OUR SPECIAL PAGES

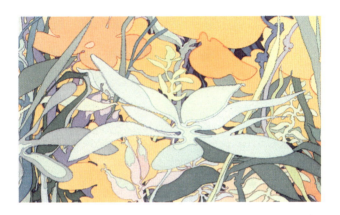

A Collection of Essays and Poems Written by Cancer Survivors

that Appeared in the Northeast Regional Cancer Institute's Newsletter,

<u>NewsNotes</u>, from 1991 to 1995.

Published by the Northeast Regional Cancer Institute
Scranton, PA

OUR SPECIAL PAGES

Cover painting: Karl Neuroth

Keystone College, La Plume, PA

Graphic design: Debra Krukowski

Condron & Co., Scranton, PA

Editor-in-chief: Susan S. Belin

Editor: Joann Scubelek

Editorial Assistant: Carrie Mohila

Acknowledgments

The Northeast Regional Cancer Institute is grateful for the thoughtful and generous contributions that made it possible to publish <u>Our Special Pages</u>:

Anonymous

Pat and John Atkins

The Family of Margaretta Belin Chamberlin

Church of the Epiphany

Bertram and Mary Ellen Linder

Forward

Life as we know it is a series of peaks and valleys. When we are in the vale it is sometimes hard to imagine making the difficult climb back to the top. The terrain may be unfamiliar and the challenges great.

We must learn to reach inside to find courage deep within our souls. As we begin the journey, one tentative step after another, we cling to the side of the mountain, being careful not to lose our footing. Forging ahead, hand over hand, we grow more determined to reach the peak, and to emerge from the shadow of the valley.

Many of us who have been fortunate to rise from the darkness into the sunlight emerge with a commitment to share the lessons we learned on our journey and to help others who are starting their ascent. The vista we see before us is miraculously clear; there is no longer a haze to cloud the beauty that surrounds us. We are filled with an appreciation for the simple things in life which many of us took for granted before we embarked on our pilgrimage.

Some of us who began the climb did not reach the summit. Their path was a difficult one, but still they persevered. We have gained strength from these courageous people, we thank them for their inspiration, and we honor their memory.

Healing thoughts and words of wisdom, humor, hope and encouragement are all to be discovered in _Our Special Pages_. No authors, by profession, will be found in this text. Just those who care to share with others their sincere and honest reflections of a time and place they have been.

Judie Harding

Our Special Pages Introduction

Our Special Pages was conceived in the hearts and minds of people who have undergone treatment for cancer. Their words of wisdom and inspiration can provide guidance and encouragement for others coping with the fears, anxieties, and stresses many people experience during their cancer diagnosis and treatment.

Our Special Pages is a compilation of writings that originally appeared in the Northeast Regional Cancer Institute's newsletter, _NewsNotes_, from 1991 through 1995. We are sincerely grateful to all these people for their willingness to share their experiences in order to help other people living with cancer, as well as their families and friends.

Some of the people who wrote their stories did not survive this devastating disease. Their words are living legacies of inspiration and courage for us all.

We especially appreciate the thoughtful contribution to _Our Special Pages_ by Karl Neuroth, director of the Department of Visual Arts at Keystone College, who donated the vibrantly colorful painting that graces the cover of the book and appears throughout the text. Karl painted this scene of his wife Scotty's flower garden when she was undergoing many months of treatment for cancer and other chronic disease. Unfortunately, Scotty died in 1991 after a long and courageous struggle.

The beauty and grace of this brilliantly alive watercolor remind us of Scotty's love of life and all of nature's bounty; the intimately intertwined flowers and leaves reflect the messages expressed in this book that love, faith, and hope are intricately woven into the delicate fabric of our lives.

We are also grateful to Debra Krukowski and Condron & Company, Inc., Scranton, who graciously and generously donated time and talent to create the handsome layout and design of _Our Special Pages_.

Most importantly, we are inspired by the thoughtful and personal works of our authors who share with us their experiences with cancer and the profound and meaningful lessons they learned about family, friends, healing, spirituality, mortality and the indomitable human spirit. We discover in *Our Special Pages* a common bond of caring and sharing in the physical and psychological struggles of people coping with cancer, learning to appreciate and embrace the precious gift of life, and living each moment and each day to the fullest:

"There is a truth I have learned from all this that is deep and profound and abiding: what we the living require most of all is each other."

"My experience made me more aware than ever of both the fragility and resilience of human life."

"I needed those tears. Tears are OK. I've learned that they wash away grief, and to grieve is important."

"As the days went by, I learned to deal with the shock, the disbelief, the denial."

"I realized how important it is to be able to give something back, and I learned to understand the real meaning of healing."

"Cancer is a lifetime battle that is not over and done with when your treatments are complete."

"It helped me translate a positive attitude into positive action."

"My experience made me more satisfied, whole and purposeful."

"What is essential is to look out on our wounded world with a heart of love; reaching out in kindness, compassion, and service."

The Northeast Regional Cancer Institute is pleased and proud to publish *Our Special Pages.*

Susan S. Belin
President

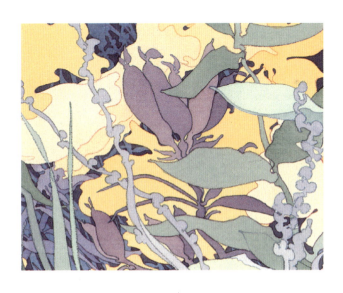

JACOB WELLER

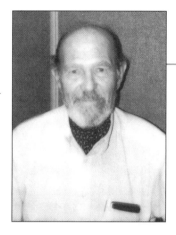

Jack Weller's vision, vitality, and commitment led to the creation of *Our Special Pages* in the Summer 1991 issue of the Northeast Regional Cancer Institute's newsletter, *NewsNotes*. Jack volunteered his time and considerable talent to serve as editor of *Our Special Pages*. His dream was to compile a book with the inspiring words and meaningful stories of cancer survivors and their care givers. To help others, Jack wrote about his personal struggles and "long voyage" through treatments for bladder cancer, and he also wrote about other survivors from whom he gained inspiration. Jack Weller died in December 1991, leaving us his legacy of *Our Special Pages*.

In Pain Deliverance

The tests were completed and the results read cancer. Suddenly everything became completely uncertain and a constant thought of death hovered about like a shadow and a fate. But I had a lot to live for, not suddenly a fate to suffer. What was I to do?

I did not have time to contemplate that, for everything happened too fast. They told me the bad news on a Wednesday and had me in the hospital the next day. X-rays, scans, tests of all kinds, and the waiting, waiting lying on my back or sitting in a wheelchair. The moments were monotonous with apprehension. I felt so vulnerable and terribly alone. Suddenly I was overwhelmed by the reality that I did not have control over my life any longer. Strangers had taken over.

This body that held my spirit had always known such good health. Now it was wracked by cancer that could very well consume me. I had dressed it, bathed it, fed it, made love with it. I had said of it, "You are me." Now I cried out in pain with it. My illusions about it had vanished. What really was this body to me? This mass of skin and bone and blood had become a stranger to me. Now I feared its sickness.

With all these thoughts running rampant in my mind I tried to put up a good front. I smiled a lot, joked with staff. It seemed to help me keep my head on an even keel, muffle the thoughts that were slowly drowning me in despair.

Now I lay in bed in agony. They had taken a big

piece of my left lung out and I had developed pneumonia along with it. And as I lay there I prayed in my own way not so much to get well as to endure... to keep my dignity, not to fall, to stand up to what I must face. And the more I thought about it the more I thought, that very well may be what life had been all about for me.

It was September and outside my hospital window a tree was slowly turning into glorious colors. The ending of the yearly cycle of birth/growth/death in Nature. Now it seemed to be my turn. But that tree somehow reassured me that all life is that way and will always begin again and again. And in that room I gazed at that tree and became very silent.

Now there are all kinds of silences. There is the silence of fear, the silence of doubt, the silence of loneliness. They are the soundless echoes of the spirit. But mine was a silence of the heart, a silence of the still, small voice within myself. The silence that enables one to know and, yes, also not to know, for isn't it best sometimes not to know? And out of that I felt a new sense of mortality, and a special affinity with people who also had suffered with cancer. I guess I should say much like the person who discovers he is alcoholic. It bound me to my fellow sufferers and changed me forever.

Then through the silence a revelation that acceptance is the thing! "God grant me the serenity to accept the things I cannot change, the courage to change the things I can, and the wisdom to know the difference," they say in Alcoholics Anonymous. And that acceptance allowed me to realize that what I felt or did would determine what the outcome would be. Right then I made a decision to let doctors and staff handle my physical problems and I could best help them heal me by trying to attain a healthy mental attitude.

So in my silence deep in the night in that hospital bed I started my feeble striving to hold onto life. And my life started to glow again in that room of waiting shadows.

But little did I know that the agony of the operations was as nothing compared to the effects of chemotherapy on my mind. It was a medicinal poison to me that made me worse so as to make me better. It insidiously caught me up in a fearful, indecisive, terribly depressed state of ennui. It made me hostile and anti-social. But the most frightening aspect was that I knew what it was doing to my brain, but I was absolutely incapable of fighting through it to stay up-beat and optimistic.

I desperately needed people and they were there. Cancer patients, some in treatment and others in remission, doctors and medical staff who had suffered through with so many before me, the American Cancer Society, friends, and almost strangers who knew of my plight, all a single infallible spirit that if I let them be my faith and hope they would pull me back to safe ground. And they did just that.

Out of what we are, out of what the world has made of us we touch, and in the touching there is a wordless, tongueless knowledge that the destinies of all living things are bound together and that what we the living require most of all is each other, and the wise man can grow wiser learning it.

I have made a long voyage and I have seen the dark side very close and there is a truth I have learned from all this that is deep and profound and abiding and yet is as simple and silent as the first word of a secret. I have learned that kindness and love can pay for an awful lot of pain and suffering.

Summer 1991

Linda's Story

by Jacob Weller

"Being a mother made me strong," said Linda Kresse as she told the story of her battle with a malignant brain tumor.

For two years she suffered with head aches, vomiting and aching eyes that couldn't stand light of any kind. It was a nightmare period when she could not function anywhere near normal. She had consulted three doctors, all of whom diagnosed her problem as migraine headaches.

One evening in March of 1988 she went deaf. Terribly frightened, she sat on her bed wondering what was really wrong with her, when suddenly her hearing returned. What was it? She went to her family doctor and told him she wasn't leaving his office until she got a specific answer to her torment. She was sent to an ear, nose, and throat specialist who discovered swelling in her inner ear. A CAT scan revealed a tumor on her brain. An appointment was made with a neurosurgeon in Philadelphia where a biopsy would be performed.

"I wanted them to get on with what they had to do so I could be a mother again. I was home the next day, which was Palm Sunday, because I wanted to share Easter a week early with my kids, knowing I'd be in the hospital for a while. Victoria was only seven months and Joseph two years at the time. Anyway, they said I should go into the hospital on Monday.

"We quickly decorated the house for the kids. Early Easter morning, which was really Palm Sunday morning, I had an egg hunt in the yard. We had to leave in the afternoon, but I had a normal Easter for my children. I kissed them good-bye and saw them standing holding their baskets waving at me.

"Monday morning the biopsy was done and it showed that the tumor was malignant. I had a rare type of cancer that's usually found only in children. Besides that, the tumor was inoperable.

"The doctor told me all this in my hospital room with my husband and family and friends there. I wanted it that way. My husband couldn't stop crying. Gee, I worried about him more than I worried about myself. I just wanted the cancer to be over with so I could be a mother and a wife again.

"I don't know why, I wasn't frightened. Being a mother and a wife I couldn't show fear. I never thought about dying. It's crazy. I don't know why. I have my beliefs...I believe in God."

So at age 24, and the mother of two small children, Linda began her fight to beat cancer. She did not have an easy time of it.

Linda had two months of radiation therapy that went from her back down her spine. "There were days when I didn't want to go for my treatment...too sick, and being so weak...but I still went.

"I'd get home from my treatment exhausted. My Joey, as little as he was, would help me get to bed. He'd say, 'Mommy, take your nap now.' He played Mommy.

"Then when it was time for his nap he'd get in my bed and twirl my hair till he fell asleep. So when I knew my hair was falling out because of the radiation I took scissors and cut my hair and put it in a bag. Joey slept with that bag and had the comfort of having Mommy's hair to twirl.

"I told Joey all that happened every step of the way. People thought I shouldn't, but I wanted him to know everything. I always told him the truth. I didn't want him to have fears about cancer.

"I was stubborn. As sick as I was I got up and made dinner for my family and then got back in bed. My mother or mother-in-law served it. I wasn't allowed to be left alone, so they stayed with me.

"And I wasn't allowed visitors because of the chance of getting an infection. Anyway, I didn't want people to see me. I really looked horrible. I remember a very hot day putting on my bathing suit...had no hair, was so thin, looked a sight. My Joey looked up at me and said, 'Oh Mommy, you look so beautiful!' I fell on my knees and hugged him.

"Oh how I wanted to be normal for my husband and children, wanted life to be the same as always. But through all that terrible time I never had the fear of dying, never thought of it. I worried about my family and never put myself first."

Then during July 1988, Linda's treatments were over and she went into remission, her dead tumor reduced to the size of a pea. All she had left were follow-up visits every three months. Her first one would be that October.

"It was Halloween, time for my first checkup and I wanted to get dressed up in a costume for the children in the hospital. The only one who knew about it was my psychological therapist. She was wonderful. I had gone to her because I had no one I could really talk to. No one in my family could handle my feelings without getting terribly upset. Anyway, I dressed up as a clown and took along 500 lollipops. I went to every child's room. To see them smile made me glow like anything. I hate to see people sad.

"Then I went back to the radiation center and got my doctor out by the desk. Had all the staff around him when I pinned a duck on him and said, 'I pinned a quack.' I think the world of him, he saved my life.

"When I was healthy enough, I got together with the American Cancer Society to be in a support group. It started for me when I met a woman who had brain cancer. I helped her pick out her wig, supported her, it was wonderful. I helped somebody. She became a close friend. Then she knew another woman with a brain tumor, so we all got in the support group.

"My first friend drifted away and wouldn't see anyone. Stayed to herself. She never made it. Only in her early 30's with two children, same as me. My family didn't tell me when she died, I guess they wanted to protect me.

"Support groups are so very important, at least to me. The more you talk about your sickness the better you feel. You get the anger out. Makes you feel better about yourself because everybody there has gone through cancer themselves, or their spouses have gone through it with them. You have to think positive, get involved with others."

Besides being a member of a support group, Linda is a volunteer driver for the American Cancer Society and she has won the Cancer Society's walk-a-thon two years in a row.

"There is life after cancer. All I want in my life with this cancer is to see my children grow, graduate and see them get married."

"I've had blessings. In May, Victoria was in her first dance recital. Her father went up on stage afterwards and presented her with three red roses. I got to see her dance. Everything I do now means much more. I've grown wiser in my early life."

And if cancer comes back? Linda said firmly, "It may come back but I'll just do it again!"

Author's Note: Yes, Linda has had blessings! She gave birth to a beautiful 7lb., 7oz. baby girl, Sophia Lynn, on August 28, 1991. Both mother and daughter are doing very well.

Linda was cautioned that she was taking a risk having another child, but to her, being pregnant was a miracle. To her, being alive was a miracle.

We congratulate Linda on such a happy occasion and thank her for sharing her story with us. We wish the entire Kresse family much health and happiness in the years to come!

Fall 1991

SR. KATHRYN BIRDSALL

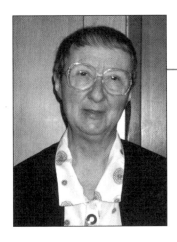

Sr. Kathryn Birdsall, IHM, entered the Congregation of the Sisters, Servants of the Immacualate Heart of Mary (IHM) in 1942, and served as an elementary school teacher for over forty years. She published a book of her poetry entitled "In Poetry We Bond" and contributed her services to the Catherine McAuley House, the Marian Convent, and the IHM Infirmary and Retirement House. Sr. Kathryn died in January 1996, "daring the leap to Love's Eternity!"

A Hair-Raising Experience

I lost my hair four times in the past decade -
a "minor" side effect of chemo and radiation,
but devastating to see Yul Brenner reflected in my mirror.

Each time, my wig was laid aside
as lacy fuzz of hair appeared
and gradually new strands expanded
to form a sparse coiffure.

This miracle of new life and growth
exploded in high hopes,
and made me feel akin to all the world's new life -
each blade of grass, tiny twig, bud and blossom.

Now, velvety lawns are mine, leafy trees,
    butterflies and birds.
Even ants are safe with me,
as the world's new life courses through my veins.

This "hair-raising" experience has
wrought great change.
    The ebb and flow,
        the come and go
            of hair four times lost
has loosened my grasp on temporalities
and "headed" me toward Infinity!

Spring 1993

Resilience

by Sr. Kathryn Birdsall, IHM

Life's marathon, a rugged race
for one too finely tuned.
"Burned out" three times
before the phrase was coined,
weakness was a bitter draught,
a vortex fathomless,
engulfing me in labyrinthine depths.

Yet, in each crisis unexpectedly arose
buoyancy, resiliency, renewed strength and wit
to glimpse humor despite distress
and bounce back to new beginnings.

Triple bouts of cancer since '82
were gifted with acceptance
and a new-found peace
as if all that went before
formed only a dissonant prelude
to a richer harmony.

Strength and courage are never my own,
for weakness has taught me there is a Source,
invisible, intangible but Real.
In womb-like suspension,
I have experienced
an Encircling Strength!

So, no "Doctor Death" for me!
Though I fear pain and what the future holds,
I trust the God of Resilience
to provide the bounce I need
for hanging in, then letting go
and daring the leap
to Love's Eternity!

Summer 1993

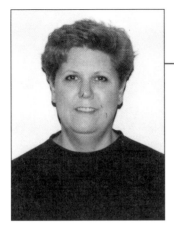

MARTHE WENTOVICH CHINDEMI

Marthe Chindemi feels a strong commitment to helping others living with cancer by offering "a little healing for the mind and soul". She works with the Patient-to-Patient support program to help ease the way for patients through the sometimes difficult physical and psychological demands of their therapy. Marthe and her daughter Elissa enjoy their time as the enthusiastic pit crew and cheering section for her husband John's NASCAR Legends car racing.

A Message of Thanks and Hope: God's Mortal Hands

Some would say 1992 was the year my life as I knew it was over. I say it was the year God began to show me the best was yet to come.

I wrote the poem, "God's Mortal Hands", as a tribute to my family doctor, Neal M. Davis, DO, who has made a profound difference in the quality of my life. Without his compassion and understanding I would not have the ability to accept the challenges God has given me. Working as a Medical Technician for twenty years, I had the opportunity to observe many physicians. I knew mine was special.

We have been through so much together in the past three years. Two hospitalizations in December 1992,

and the diagnosis of multiple sclerosis. Two operations in April 1994 for endometrial cancer, and the summer spent in radiation therapy. Through it all he was there for me. I would come in upset for many appointments, and he would sit back, put his feet up, and let me get it all out. He understood how difficult all this was both physically and emotionally for me. When I was done we would talk it through.

Because of the multiple sclerosis I had to resign from my job, but I am thankful for my medical background. I researched my illnesses as much as possible, sitting in bookstores and libraries for hours and hours to learn all I could. Then I would share my questions and concerns with Dr. Davis. He would listen and we would discuss the best alternatives. It reminded me of a flea market: I would try to get the painful aspects reduced to minimum, and we would bargain back and forth and end up with an acceptable compromise. He never took exception to my suggestions. It was therapy for me to be so actively involved in my care, and he continues to encourage it.

That is why I sat down a few days before Christmas last year and thought about what special gift I could give him to express my gratefulness. I have never written poetry, nor had I even cared to read it. The words seemed to come from nowhere. (I guess I should say they came from God's inspiration.)

I wanted to incorporate in my words to Dr. Davis a message to all patients, and to share the thoughts and feelings that helped me through the rough times. God has given us prayer, doctors, friends and family to help us through. Use them all!

I have never once said "Why me?" I am no better than anyone else. Sometimes it takes adversity to make us aware of all our blessings.

My life has changed for the better through all of this. I have become sensitive to the many things I had taken for granted or never noticed. I received help, prayers, and concern from people I never knew cared so much. I never would have known how loving and good my husband John could be. My daughter Elissa did all the laundry, and took care of me while I was in bed recovering, and never once complained. I used to feel guilty about being sick and not able to do the things I should to take care of them. Elissa was only seven when all this started, but she was happy to do it. Even when I was better, she still wanted to help.

Please remember you too can get through whatever obstacles come your way. Take the time to discover all your options and give it all you've got. And when it's all over you will feel so good. It's like running a marathon, long and hard. You will feel so much joy and accomplishment when it's over. You will be a new person and will never take anything for granted again.

I thank all my physicians, nurses, radiation technologists, and others who helped in my care. Their job is a difficult one. They work with us cancer patients everyday and deal with our despair, yet they always have a smile on their faces and a kind word.

I am looking forward to my first Cancer Survivors Day and to the rest of my life.

God's Mortal Hands

The treatments seemed unbearable
I stopped them out of fear; I prayed to God to heal me
I thought He did not hear
So when I died I asked Him "Why?"
"My Child I Gave You Doctors, To Save Your Life So Dear"
I then awoke and was glad to find
My death was just a dream
He sent his message in my sleep
"We Three Must Be A Team"
Now I know what I must do; In order for me to heal
And I thank the Lord every day
For sending Dr. Neal

Summer 1995

RUSS COLLINS & LYNNY SIEGAL

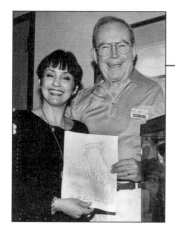

Russ Collins and Lynny Siegal work as a team to share their message of hope with people undergoing cancer treatment. Speaking from their different personal experiences with cancer, they offer helping hands and encouraging words to patients who are undergoing radiation therapy.

Don't Ever Giver Up!

It has been almost 36 months since I was first diagnosed with colon cancer. After an operation and many sessions of radiation and chemotherapy, I discovered that my original cancer had spread to my liver. In December of 1992, I underwent my second cancer operation.

I wish that I could speak to all cancer patients to tell them how wonderful I feel today and to encourage them to be very positive in their outlook for recovery. Because I have experienced fear, anxiety, physical pain and discomfort, I decided I might help other patients in a personal way. I try to spend every Tuesday in the radiation oncology department and in the inpatient oncology unit at Mercy Hospital, Scranton.

I usually begin with: "Hi! My name is Russ Collins. I am a two time survivor and I would like to talk with you for a few minutes. First I want to give you one of my famous pictures of the Heron and the Frog. Look at it closely and then read what it says at the bottom of the page: 'Don't ever give up!' That should be the motto of us cancer survivors."

That is my opening "spiel", and 99 percent of the time it is well received. Then we go upstairs to visit the inpatients. There, Lynny Siegal, my co-volunteer and the person whom I call my "boss," introduces us. "Hi. I'm Lynny, and this is Russ. We are volunteers and we would like to visit with you for a few minutes."

Lynny is the mother of a cancer survivor. Her son was diagnosed at age 11 with lymphoma. Today he is a young man of 24, and leads a full and normal life in every way.

Lynny and I share a common goal to show cancer patients that there is life after hearing those dreaded words from the doctor: "I'm afraid it is malignant." To many people, including friends and caretakers as well as patients, that pronouncement is seen as a certain death sentence. We want to show them that this is not necessarily so. Remission and cure are possible. Through a positive mental attitude, lots of faith, great support from family and friends, excellent doctors and nurses, and services available at our area hospitals, this terrible disease can be beaten in so many more cases than ever before. *"Don't ever give up!"*

As a mother, caretaker, faithful volunteer, and my special friend Lynny explains: "Laughter is the best medicine. Being the mother of a cancer survivor, I cannot relate to the same pain, fatigue, and fear that the patients experience. However, I know the pain, the heartache, and the fatigue one feels from watching a loved one suffer, and of course the fear and worry about the future.

"The helplessness many family members or caretakers experience is overwhelming, especially when your loved one is feeling 'lousy.'

"I can relate to the person left sitting on those chairs in the waiting areas, wondering how the person will be feeling after treatment. A sense of humor, faith, and strength of mind helps keep caretakers going. Those volunteers who appear with a smile and a touch when they are needed help the time pass a little faster.

"I watch my fellow volunteer and good friend Russ with patients in radiation oncology and when we visit patients in the oncology unit. I see how his smile, his famous picture and his special touch make their day a little brighter. We work together every Tuesday and complement each other's style. We both enjoy laughter ~ a very important component of our volunteer jobs and the cancer patients' road to recovery. We almost always leave them smiling."

We can't call what we do "work." It is an opportunity to "give something back." We are the fortunate ones whose mental attitude, prayers of family and friends, caring doctors, nurses and technicians made it possible for us to be survivors. God bless them!

We recognize that too many people have fought the good fight, only to succumb to cancer, and we honor and remember their courage. Our mission is to tell that many people have survived to live normal, healthy, and happy years.

Above all, we want to end this article by repeating our motto and slogan: *"Cancer patients: Don't ever give up!!!"*

Summer 1994

JOAN DAVIS

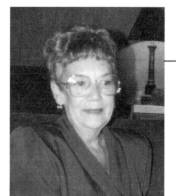

Joan Davis credits her good friends, great doctors, and caring husband Ron for the glorious nine years she has enjoyed since her cancer treatment. "God willing," she says, "I'm taking them all with me into the 21st century!" Joan works to help others living with cancer as a volunteer with the Patient-to-Patient Program at Mercy Hospital, Scranton.

Thanks for These Glorious Years!

"Hey God! It's me again, Joanie the pest." This is how I end each and every evening, thanking HIM for another day.

Eight and a half years ago I was diagnosed with ovarian cancer. Stage III-C, metastasized to the colon in two locations. Two days after surgery my doctors informed me of my condition. I shocked myself by handling this devastating news so well, or perhaps I was in denial. My prognosis was not very promising. I left the oncologist's office with the intention of "putting my house in order" so to speak.

On the same day my brother and only sibling was diagnosed with lung cancer. "This couldn't be happening to us!" When reality set in, I knew we had a difficult road ahead. My brother, for reasons we do not know, refused surgery and treatment. He died two years later.

I received eight months of aggressive chemotherapy, each treatment lasting forty eight hours. I was one sick Cookie! I weighed eighty pounds and looked dreadful. I was convinced I would never see Christmas. I refused to purchase a pair of much needed shoes because I would never get the chance to wear them. Well, nine Christmas trees and at least thirty pair of shoes later, I'm still going strong!

I won't pretend this was all a breeze... it's not easy for any of us. I had some very trying times. But I was lucky, I had my husband Ron and I knew he was there for me. He cooked, cleaned the house and took very good care of me. While I must confess that some of those microwave meals were not very palatable... I'm thankful he was there! !

If any one were to ask what helped the most, I would have to say getting involved! Ron and I joined cancer groups. He learned all there was to know about ovarian cancer, I only went along for the ride. But before I knew it, I was actually looking forward to these meetings.

We belong to "Couples Facing Cancer", a support group held each Tuesday evening at Mercy Hospital in Scranton.

As a trained volunteer for the American Cancer Society's "Can Surmount" program, I speak with newly diagnosed cancer patients. I'd like to think I've helped some of them because I know helping them has helped me! I feel really good when I know I've put a patient's mind at ease... I know where they are coming from because I've been there.

There isn't a day goes by that I don't think about cancer... But I can promise each and every one of you newly diagnosed friends reading this... it does get easier... much easier. Don't put yourselves through the "I'm going to die syndrome" as I did. Have faith! ! !

Well, it's that time of night again... I've brushed my teeth, put on my P.J.'s and am all ready to hop into bed.

"Hey, God! It's me again, Joanie the pest. Just wanted to check in with you and say thanks for these glorious eight and half years. I know the next eight and a half years will be even better... AMEN! ! ! !"

Spring 1995

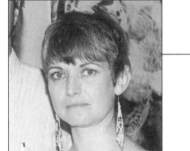

SHARON DeNAULT

Sharon DeNault, BFA, MAT, completed her Masters Degree in Art Therapy in 1995, 13 years after her treatment for breast cancer. She finds painting and sculpting personally therapeutic, and now works as an art therapist at Allied Services to help people coping with chronic disease learn to relax and enjoy the creative process. Sharon takes daily chemotherapy medication for a rare form of blood cancer.

An Invitation to a Cancer Party!

Ten years ago, this spring, someone invited me to a "cancer party." Unfortunately, it was an invitation I couldn't refuse.

I bravely put on my "party mask" as so many cancer patients do, and pretended everything was A-OK. I had entered a classic state of denial.

My timing was "the pits" as my husband so eloquently told me. He was busy with our new business while I was supplying the only reliable income at the time. Fortunately, I had the support of my wonderful mother and my family. Later there would be a whole new group of friends I met through *Reach to Recovery*.

Those early months I handled with such

strength, or so I thought. What I heard from everyone was "what a great attitude you have." That's because I was continually laughing and making fun of all the things so many others cry about.

I worked with the American Cancer Society *Reach to Recovery* program for several years after my mastectomy. It was after working with one family in particular that I finally confronted the unresolved issues concerning my mastectomy. One day the husband asked me to come to his office to talk. He wanted to know what he could do for his cancer-stricken wife. How could he help her adjust? Showing his sincere concern, he shared with me his fear of losing her, and his shame for feeling helpless when she appeared so brave.

As I left his office I was traumatized by the realization of my own denial. The denial of my deepest fear of dying and my sincere need to be nurtured.

I reached my car, looked at the road in front of me, held tightly to the steering wheel, and for the first time since my surgery two years before, I cried. I cried for the fact that I never had that kind of support; my husband dealt with my cancer by finding another woman. I cried for the fact that I was tired of acting so together. I cried for the fact that I was afraid to leave my marriage. What could I do on my own?

I needed those tears. Tears are okay. I've learned that they wash away grief, and to grieve is important.

Swallowing my pride, I called one of my doctors. From previous experiences I knew he would be objective, concerned, and focused. I told him what I was living with in my marriage, or rather living without. We decided I needed to find something to compensate for the lack of understanding in my marriage and to help me find some answers to the difficult questions I was wrestling with at that time.

The solution: a clean sheet of paper! My task was to paint my future.

Always a frustrated artist, I signed up for the first available oil painting class. All those feelings that I was afraid to face came out on the canvas. As I healed myself through art, my self-esteem flourished.

Ten years after my surgery... divorced, still a mother of two (a daughter engaged to be married and a son in fifth grade), a senior at Marywood College in Art, and soon to pursue my Master's Degree in Art Therapy.

It's important to me to be able to relate to others what I've learned about gaining control of our lives. Through the many forms of art, such as poetry, music, writing, painting, sculpting, drama, and dance we can discover our fears and frustrations and release them.

Through creativity we have the power to create our own kind of life. There should be at least one medium that can open a door to the inner person for everyone. Art has made such a difference in my healing, that I'm now on a personal mission to include art in every cancer patient's genre for living.

Summer 1992

LORRAINE FOSTER

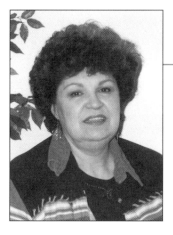

Lorraine Foster is always happy to relate to others how helpful it was for her to discover and utilize the power of the mind/body connection to reduce stress, relieve pain, and instill a positive outlook while dealing with her cancer diagnosis and treatment. Lorraine says she continues to practice daily relaxation and visualization techniques to keep her healthy, happy, and cancer-free.

Calling on the Healer Within

Hello, my name is Lorraine Foster. . . and I am a cancer survivor.

After my yearly mammogram in early 1992, I received a phone call to return for additional x-rays, "Suspicious shadow," What is that? Cancer, surgery, disfigurement, death? All these things crossed my mind as I waited to hear the diagnosis from my physician. "Cancer," He said it . . . and I went numb.

Being the logically minded person that I am, I decided not to get hysterical just then. I would save it until later, just in case I would really need it. I stayed calm and was able to discuss my options and care plan with my doctors.

I also made up my mind that this cancer was not going to conquer me... I was going to conquer it. But while acting bravely on the outside, the worry and concern were mounting on the inside. I knew it was time to use my mind-body connection to get me through what lay ahead.

Hypnosis! That was my plan. I have a very special friend, Jeanne, who is an internationally certified professional hypnosis therapist and counselor. Having complete confidence in her as a specialist in her field, I was able to relax and concentrate on learning how to use hypnosis to cope with all of the physical and emotional symptoms of my illness.

It took very little time for Jeanne to teach me how to trigger my relaxation response and I was able to use these techniques throughout my diagnostic tests and biopsy surgery. When a lumpectomy was indicated, I once again turned to hypnosis.

With permission from my doctor and the anesthetist, I became the first patient at the hospital I chose to be hypnotized in the pre-surgical area. I went into surgery free of all anxiety and completely relaxed. It was almost amusing when they had to wake me up in order to put me to sleep for the procedure.

Pain management was also part of Jeanne's program for me. I was able to perform the post-surgical exercises easily and control any discomfort during my radiation and chemotherapy treatments in the following months. I continue to use hypnosis as a healing tool in my life. I will continue to seek Jeanne's help as I continue to **survive**.

Since my encounter with breast cancer, I now look at life differently. Eyes that before only looked, now see; and ears that only heard, now listen. I thank God for the very qualified physicians, caring nurses, and the special love and support of family and friends. Because I received so much from so many people, I hope to turn a negative situation into a positive one by sharing my experience with relaxation therapy with other women also facing the uncertainty of breast cancer.

Jeanne's Perspective:

Lorraine used several simple techniques involving visualization, imagery, and deep breathing in order to keep her thoughts focused. By reducing the stress and anxiety of her physical self, she was able to remain calm and relaxed through all procedures.

While in the hypnotic state, Lorraine was able to open her subconscious mind and became more receptive to the suggestions that her body was getting well.

Suggestions that she was given under hypnosis for relaxation, a positive attitude, and pain control were later triggered by a finger touch and a special word. Whenever she used these techniques, the positive affirmations were reinforced in her mind and became her dominant thought, thus allowing her body to react in the same direction as that thought.

The time it takes to develop these techniques varies from person to person, but Lorraine and I found it well worth the time and effort for the benefits of restored health. Remember, personal rewards are equal to personal endeavors.

Lorraine and I appreciate the understanding and support of many in our medical community for allowing hypnosis therapy to be used as a part of a team approach for improved health care.

We sincerely hope that we can help guide other people to their own inborn ability to connect their mind and body to aid the healing process.

NRCI Editor's Note: Hypnosis therapy can be adjunct therapies to minimize the side effects of cancer treatment. However, it does not replace conventional medical treatment.

Winter 1994

SHAWN GIPSON

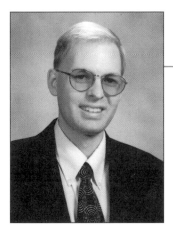

Shawn Gipson suffered a second bout with cancer in the winter of 1996, but he again fought successsfully to overcome his disease. He is now a second year college student in Arkansas, and is even more determined "with hope and flare . . . to win a grand."

Sonnet #1

Just when you think your life couldn't get worse,
Murphy's Law takes over and things go wrong.
You are feeling bad, as sick as a horse,
That horse, now weak, was once virile and strong.

A Golden Palomino I once was,
Until Cancer took me out of the race.
A horse with a bum leg can't run because,
Three instead of four is too slow a pace.

I fight and fight to regain my strength,
Three weeks on, three weeks off, is all I got.
Like a horse trying to run just one length,
With Work and Love, I have only one shot.

When my treatment is all over and done,
I might look back and say "That was sure fun!"

Summer 1993

Sonnet #2

by Shawn Gibson

I was once a lover not a fighter
Giving my love to family and mankind.
Unlike Tyson who was a great fighter
Trying to block, jab and holes he must find.

A boxer must learn to punch and dodge
His first test of strength another man.
A tumor in my head had found it's lodge
Turning me from a lover with span.

Fighting cancer with a coach and her bone
I want and need to defeat this "known stand"
Into the struggle I am fully thrown
With hope and flare I want to win a grand.

After beating Tyson the world will see
In the end I wish a lover to be.

Summer 1993

JUDIE HARDING

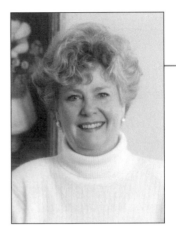

Judie Harding, a breast cancer survivor, is thankful to God, good medical care, and a wonderful support system of family and friends for helping her survive. "Life is beautiful!" says Judie, who has been married to her best friend Tom for 35 years and enjoys their three wonderful sons, three beautiful daughters-in-law, and two handsome grandsons. Her many hobbies include painting, writing, jewelry making, and snorkeling. Judie generously shares her time and talents as a volunteer ~ helping, encouraging, and inspiring other cancer survivors.

Geez, You're Looking Good!

I crawl into bed tired, but satisfied with the busy day that has just ended for me. Pulling up the covers I think about all the preparation I've done for Thanksgiving, the day after tomorrow. Today I picked up the turkey at Pallman's farm, did the grocery shopping, bought the wine and flowers. Tomorrow will be an "in-house" day, setting the dining room table in all its holiday finery, arranging flowers and cooking some of the many dishes we "must have" to make it a traditional Thanksgiving.

But now it's time for much deserved sleep. Kissing my husband good night I roll over on my right side throwing my left arm over my chest with my left hand coming to rest on my right breast. There it is ~ under my fingertips I feel a small, hard lump. It can't be! I have done self examination on a regular basis and have never felt anything out of the ordinary. A sense of panic courses through my whole body ~ my mind says, "stop it!" ~ this can't be anything serious. But my gut feeling is not a good one.

A few agonizing moments go by before I can roll over and tell my husband Tom what I have just discovered. I ask him to feel it, he does. It is also foreign to him. I try my best not to panic. After all, most lumps are not malignant, and there is no history of breast cancer in my family. Tomorrow will be a busy day so I'll put this on hold until Friday, the day after Thanksgiving.

Sleep does not come easily. I toss and turn and

think and pray. Morning dawns and I go ahead with my regular routine, although my heart is heavy and my mind will not rest.

We have family and friends for a lovely Thanksgiving day dinner. But, I must admit that deep inside I am thankful the holiday is coming to an end. I want to make arrangements to see my gynecologist.

Bright and early Friday morning I call, but the gynecologist's office is closed for the holiday weekend. I wait until Monday and call again. I get an appointment, but not for two weeks! I make another call to have a mammogram done as soon as possible, but that must wait two weeks also. Both appointments are scheduled for the same day; have the mammogram first, then see the doctor. I'm not sure how I will get through the next two weeks.

Finally, the appointed day arrives. The mammogram machine whirs away and so does my brain. Next I'm off to see the doctor, who is a friend. After examining the lump he is hopeful it is a cyst. He asks me to sit in his office while he tracks down the mammogram and has it read. He gets the call back and says to me, "You just got your first Christmas present. It's a cyst. Go on home."

I thank him for everything and walk out of there feeling as light as a feather, almost giddy.

Three days later as I am decorating for Christmas the phone rings. It is my doctor. He tells me he just got the written report on my mammogram and doesn't like what he is reading. "You had better see a surgeon." My knees buckle and I feel sick. Here we go again.

I call my husband. We talk, I cry, he comforts. Every part of me wants to scream, but I do make that call to the surgeon. First available appointment is the day after Christmas. Can I survive that long? How will I make it through another holiday?

The surgeon was a college classmate of my husband, and has a fine reputation. I feel confident that I am in good hands. He checks the lump. He does a needle aspiration, but not with good results. He says we have to do an open biopsy in the hospital on December 28th. My heart is pounding. I feel vulnerable. **Wait!** I need time to think. I tell him I'll call him in a couple of hours.

My husband is waiting for me. I cry again. Can this be happening? I call the surgeon and agree to the date for the surgical procedure.

The 28th comes; I have the biopsy. It is malignant. Now it's time to talk about my options.

I have another meeting with the surgeon to discuss my mastectomy. I set up an appointment with an oncologist. He is the same doctor who took care of my dad. My dad called him the doctor with two hearts, because "No one could be that kind and have only one heart!" My pathologist is also a friend who helps answer many of my questions.

I feel fortunate to have so many fine doctors in my corner.

I study, read, ask questions. Finally the surgery is set for January 19th. The date originally selected was January 12th, but my father died of prostate cancer in the same hospital, on that same date, so I need to postpone for a week "for me."

Surgery day I am surrounded by a loving family and supportive friends. My fine medical team includes a high school buddy who is a recovery room nurse. She holds my hand on the way to the O.R. and wishes me well.

Surgery is over, my right breast gone, and hopefully, so is all the cancer. But we'll have to wait for the pathology reports. They arrive several days later – two lymph nodes are positive.

My room is filled with flowers and many visitors come and go, each of them telling me how well I look. Funny, I don't get that feeling when I look in the mirror. Oh well!

At the end of the week, still a bit weak, I'm discharged. It's good to be home! Family and more friends and neighbors come to visit, each in his or her turn telling me how well I look.

Two days later I put on a loose top, prop a small pillow under my arm, and go to a neighbor's Super Bowl Party. Everyone says... "Geez you're looking good!"

A month goes by, I'm healing very nicely. Time to start my chemotherapy. I'm trying to be **very** positive.

I have my first treatment, and experience some side effects. I have flushed skin and nausea, and I'm tired. Nothing I can't handle. About ten days go by and my hair starts falling out. Three days later it's all gone. What a blow to the old ego. First, half of my chest, now all of my hair. I put on my wig and everywhere l go people say ... "Geez you're looking good!" (Wish they could see me without this wig.)

Another treatment and I lose my eyelashes, most of my eyebrows, plus my body hair. I look like an egg, yet from all corners I hear the same thing ... "Geez you're looking good!" (Must be the big earrings.)

It's been two years, I've got all my hair, eyebrows, and eyelashes, plus about 20 to 25 extra pounds. And from physicians, technicians, family and friends the refrain is still the same... "Geez you're looking good!"

My dad told me that there are three stages of life ~ youth, middle age, and... "Geez you're looking good!" I pray that I'm not in the "Geez" stage yet, so if you happen to see me, please tell me I look **middle age**!!!!

Summer 1992

Mask

by Judie Harding

The you you are
And the you they see
Are not always quite the same
They can be two different people
Sharing a common name.
The face put on for all the world
Belies what's deep inside
Chin thrust out with such resolve
Determined to keep your pride.
Putting up a good front
Is taught from early years
Still can't remember how or when
You learn to deal with fears.
Maybe its time to lower your guard
And peel away the mask
Put the true you in front of the world
But. . . is this wise you may ask?
Oh yes! . . . will be the answer
Think of how "special" you are
Not another around just like you
Your true self is best by far.

Spring 1995

Why Wait?

by Judie Harding

Bid yourself a good day

Honor who you are

Listen to those feelings

Make a wish on a star

Grant yourself time to do

Those things you've set aside

Joyful little pleasures

That fill your heart with pride

In giving yourself time each day

The rewards will be many fold

Perhaps you'll accomplish all your dreams

Before you grow too old.

Spring 1995

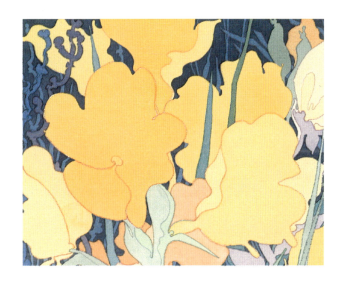

Turning Point

by Judie Harding

Four years ago Thanksgiving,
My life took a sudden turn.
Cancer was the diagnosis,
And I had much to learn.
I went from doctor to surgeon,
Then to the oncologist,
Keeping my wits about me,
There was nothing that I missed.
They did scans, tests and x-rays,
I was scared and in a daze.
Times of sorrow and triumph,
Some memories are a haze.
Next came surgery and chemo,
Lost my breast and then my hair,
There were times I was hopeful,
Other days it didn't seem fair.
Will I ever be the same again?
I wonder to myself out loud,
Will the sunshine come back to me
And chase away this cloud?
Family and friends were there for me,
I know that I am blessed
God in his infinite wisdom
Is giving me a test.
He sent me this little cross to bear,
And carry it I will,

For I have some footsteps to follow,
Even though his path was up hill
You see, Dad had cancer before me,
His burden was never light,
But he had a wonderful attitude,
As he continued his fight.
Although he lost the battle,
And we miss him every day,
He left an example to follow,
It helps me find the way.
As I walk down this path of life,
His courage is my guide,
He makes each step easier,
Cause I feel him by my side.
My wish for those who follow,
Is easy enough to state,
Enjoy each precious day of life,
And remember it's never "too late."
Take time to enjoy the little things,
Dainty flowers, trees, birds that sing,
Love your family and
embrace your friends,
Don't fail to make amends.
Be kind to yourself and you will see,
The best in life is yet to be.

Summer 1994

Cancer - You Have Taught Me

by Judie Harding

To marvel at every sunrise

To rejoice in every sunset

To take a little time for myself each day

To reach out to others

To say "I love you" more often

To cherish my family for what they are

and who they are

To be strengthened by my faith

To learn from past mistakes

Not to save anything for good - the "good times" are now

To take more chances without undue risk

To spend more time with small children

~ they are life's treasures

To appreciate my hair

To strive at making each day better than the last

To realize my personal strengths

To work at overcoming my weaknesses

To take the high road

To develop my creativity

Not to love anything that can't love me back

To truly value old friends

To embrace new friends

To listen to the messages from my body

To open all of my senses to the beauty of nature

To be a partner with my doctors

To continue setting new goals

To borrow from the strengths of others

To keep stress at bay

Not to expect flowers if I don't plant a garden

To communicate directly with others

To savor the flavor of a summer tomato

To accept my body as it is

To recognize that I can't fix everything

To live with uncertainty and expect the unexpected

To face my own mortality

To thank God for each precious day.

Winter 1994

It's PDS Time Again

by Judie Harding

My fingertips make the familiar trip down both sides of my neck, continuing over my chest and glide around to the underarm area. Feels OK! No lumps or bumps. The biggest lump I feel is in my throat. All my senses are heightened; its PDS time again: Pre-Doctor Syndrome.

This is a very familiar pattern for cancer patients ~ checking and feeling things we should, but also things we are not really qualified or trained to do. Because it is my body and I am more familiar with it than anyone else, I feel compelled to examine whatever I can.

PDS can last from several days to several weeks, and affects different people in different ways. For me it can be a vague, empty feeling or a frightening rush of adrenaline when I feel a twinge in my back, or a pain in my belly. I am sure this is a signal that the cancer has metastasized, rarely taking into account that these aches and pains could be from carrying that heavy package, or gas pains from all those peanuts I indulged in.

Our minds play tricks that can frighten us more than the boogie man. Even the most rational of us allows little doubts to creep into our minds at times, making us less than pleasant to be around.

It is sometimes very hard to explain to our loved ones and friends that a minor complaint has sent us into a tizzy. Try as you may, it's not always easy to chase those doubts away.

The experts tell us to keep stress out of our lives. I wonder how many of them have tried meditation or visualization while having a bone scan, CAT scan, MRI, or whatever. Your main focus at that time is on the results of the test ~ and if you are a religious person, you are probably very busy making deals with God. PDS brings back these moments of stress.

D-Day (Doctor Day) is here. You do the necessary preparation to look your best and clutch the list of questions you have prepared. You arrive at the appointed hour, sign in, and find a seat in the waiting room. Every now and then there is a familiar face. You greet each other, exchanging pleasantries. You pick up a magazine, but rarely get into anything that requires a lot of concentration. Instead, you leaf through the pages and glance around the waiting room wondering about the other patients ~ or are they care givers? Many times it's hard to tell.

The door opens, your name is called. You go into the room beyond to be greeted by the smiling faces of the nurses and technicians who always seem happy to see you. You take a seat, a rubber tourniquet is put on your arm and you pray today will be the day when the necessary blood samples can be drawn on the first attempt. It's not easy, especially after chemotherapy has left those veins less cooperative. Ahh, success and on the first try! Now it's back to the waiting room. Your name is called again, and you are on your way to the examining room.

But, first there's a stop at the dreaded scale. Each visit I fantasize that the scale is broken and out for repair. No such luck. I set my purse on the chair, slip out of my shoes and slowly get on the scale. Next time I must remember to wear a silk outfit that weighs next to nothing. As the weights are moved into position, I vow I will weigh ten pounds less by the next visit.

On to the examining room. Blood pressure is taken and noted. It's time to disrobe and put on that beautiful couturier creation called a hospital gown. Did you ever wonder why you took the time to select a snazzy outfit when all your doctor will see is the same style blue green-gown he saw on the patient before? Oh, well!

I boost myself up on the examining table and wait. This is the time I am alone with my thoughts. It's a time to reflect on the wintry days that have passed and ponder the future that lies ahead. Before long the door opens and the doctor enters with a big "Hello!" Immediately he inquires about how I am feeling. I fill him in on what's been going on since the last visit. Time for the examination. As his fingers skillfully probe the areas I have already checked, I pray he won't find any abnormalities. Just a few minutes can seem like an eternity.

Examination complete and all systems are go. WHEW! Made it through one more time. That wasn't so bad. The tightness in my throat is easing and the heaviness in my chest is lifting.

Sitting up, I remember my list of questions. Some are very valid, others seem more trivial. All are important to give me the information I need, or to ease my mind. The doctor answers my questions and helps allay some of my fears. I wish he had a crystal ball and we could know the future. But then reality kicks in and I remember that each day we have is a very precious gift, and I am grateful for every one.

This is certainly one of the benefits of being a cancer survivor. . . knowing just how precious life is. If only we could impart this special feeling to those who take so many little things for granted.

The doctor finishes writing on my chart, bids me a good day, and is off to see the patient in the next room. You know, the one in the same blue-green gown and sweaty palms, with a different list of questions.

I hop down from the examining table, get dressed, and proceed to the office to make my next appointment ~ and take care of my bill!

Driving home, I think about how fortunate I am to have access to top quality medical care, to be free to choose my doctor, hospital, and even course of treatment. Yes, I am truly blessed in many ways.

I will have about ten weeks free from PDS, and then as the time draws nearer for my next appointment, my mind will start working over time and my fingers will check for lumps and bumps. But, next time I will retread these thoughts I have put on paper, take a deep breath, think positive thoughts, and thank God for all the time I have to keep my doctor's appointments.

Summer 1992

Cancer Victim

by Judie Harding

C   *Courage to face whatever may be*

A   *Attitude ~ it's important*

N   *Never take life for granted*

C   *Commitment to help other survivors*

E   *Educate myself and others about this disease*

R   *Relax and enjoy life*

V   *Victor each day that I am here*

I   *Insight to know what is important*

C   *Comedy ~ Laughter is the best medicine*

T   *Thankfulness for the support of family and friends*

I   *Interest in all that is around me*

M   *Motivation to accept new challenges*

Don't count me out just yet! I don't deserve your pity, for I have been on a journey that has taken me to highs and lows like I have never known...but I am here and I still feel...good and bad, happy and sad...just like you.

We are all terminal, I've had a reminder of my mortality...some are never fortunate enough to be given the chance to say "I love you" with such ease, to look at nature with renewed appreciation, to make amends for "whatever".

I have been blessed in many ways. If you had to choose a path, which one would it be? A sudden heart attack, an accident, a stroke ~ just a few of the many paths we might have to walk ~ some easier than others, but each with its peaks and valleys.

Cancer is just one of the many avenues to the end of this part of our journey.

My plan is to take a slow walk down the road of life as we know it here on earth. Hopefully to live to be an old woman who is much wiser and can share that wisdom with all those who thought of her as a victim, when in reality she was one of the millions of cancer patients or survivors on the road to......
THE END!

Author's Note: While I am deeply grateful to the press for all the coverage given to cancer-related issues, in too many instances the person in the article is referred to as a cancer "victim". It is my hope that in the future this will be changed to "patient", "survivor", or "victor".

Fall 1994

ELLEN HOLMAN

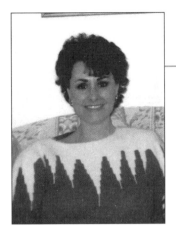

Ellen Holman, an eight-year survivor of Hodgkin's disease, has shared her valuable time and advice in a variety of ways to help people who are undergoing cancer treatment. A former special education teacher, Ellen now keeps busy enjoying her volunteer work, her husband Don, and their two children: 21-year old Kim and 15-year old Jennifer.

How Can You Help a Person With Cancer?

Listen! Being a good listener is the most important quality you need to help a person with cancer. Cancer patients need to tell "their story", pouring out their anxiety and concerns.

The listener must be sincere, caring, and truly concerned about the person. Cancer survivors who are in remission can be excellent "listeners" because they can share similar feelings and experiences. So many people coping with cancer have said to me "it was great to have someone listen to me so I could get this off my chest".

Encouragement is also important to help people cope with their illness. They want to hear your story and how long you have been in remission. Be truthful about your surgery, chemotherapy, or radiation therapy, but always try to encourage and be positive. We all encounter set backs and side effects during our treatment, but it is not helpful to offer details of some of your not-so-pleasant experiences! Encourage the person to be positive and take one day at a time.

I will never forget the people who encouraged me through my illness. They will always be a very special part of my memory and my life.

There are so many little things we can do for people with cancer. Take the time to make a phone call or send a card with an encouraging note. A surprise in the mail is always a pick-me-up. Send a small book of poems, a humorous book, or a book of short stories. A basket of fruit or a bouquet of flowers are always welcome.

A friendly visit can be especially helpful and most appreciated. Bring along a small house plant, an apple pie, cookies, or a few groceries. Cancer patients have good days and bad days, so always call before you visit. I remember being caught off guard a few times and answering the door with a bald head or a wig on sideways. However, it was always nice to know that others cared, and their visits helped make my days a little easier.

Another way to help is to provide a home-cooked meal. It needn't be fancy. If they can't use the meal that day, they can put it in the freezer until they really need it. If possible, try to set up a few weeks of meals for people with the help of their friends, family, and neighbors. When they feel well enough, invite them out to lunch or to your home for supper.

Meals are always a worry for people undergoing cancer treatment, especially when they have a family to take care of. When I received two months of radiation treatments, people from my church brought meals every day. It was such a burden lifted from my shoulders to know that my family was taken care of during those difficult days until I got back on my feet. These special people will always be dear to me for being there when I really needed them.

Energy levels can get very low during treatment, and having help with daily household chores can be a great benefit. Offer to run the vacuum, dust, clean the bathroom, put a few loads in the washer or dryer or fold the wash. I remember how difficult it was for me to carry the baskets of laundry down the cellar steps. It took all the energy I had to get the heavy load back up the steps and put away. The little tasks most of us do routinely each day can be very difficult and exhausting for a person undergoing cancer treatment.

For younger patients, offer to take the children for a few hours. Give the parent a chance to take a bubble bath, read a book, take a nap or a walk. People on treatment get very little time for themselves. They spend so much of their time and energy at the doctor's office, or getting blood work or X-rays. Give them the time they need and deserve. It may be the best gift you can give.

Another wonderful way to help is to offer to drive for radiation or chemotherapy treatments. It is always nice to have company along for the ride, as well as to have someone to talk with while waiting for treatment. Having a friend along helps relieve the anxiety. I always had someone drive me for my treatments. By being with me, they helped to share some of the pain and that made the day easier for me.

If you can try just a few of these suggestions, you can make a cancer patient's day so much brighter. Just knowing that people care about you and are willing to share their love in these small ways helps us to get through treatments. By making a small difference in a cancer patient's day, you will make a large difference in their quality of life.

Winter 1995

Thank You For Those Little Things That Mean So Much

by Ellen Holman

To our doctors, nurses and technicians:

Thank you for giving me a smile when I may feel the whole world is caving in on me or just may not feel well that day. Whether I am sitting in a doctor's office, having blood taken, waiting to have x-rays taken or lying on a gurney ~ I need your smile. Your "special smile" can turn the whole day around and bring some sunshine into a cloudy day.

Thank you for listening to me and answering my questions. It makes me feel good to know that my comments and concerns are as important to you as they are to me. I appreciate doctors speaking to me in terms that I can understand and taking the time to explain medical terms that need explaining.

Thank you for telling me how wonderful I look ~ even though I have lost my hair, or lost or gained weight. While undergoing treatments, we may not have many days when we feel we look good. It means so much to us when you say we do!

Thank you for calling me as quickly as possible when lab reports or x-ray results arrive. We seem to have so much waiting, and being a patient does not seem to get easier. A few days can I seem like weeks. How special it can be to share good reports ~ not just the bad ones!

Thank you for laughing with me. I may suffer emotional or physical pain, but I still need to laugh. I appreciate doctors, nurses, and technicians who can sandwich some humor in-between those layers of hurt and pain. It helps to laugh at our hair falling out or the knobby knees on the guy in the hospital gown.

Thank you for making me feel that I am a very important person. Thank you for asking me how I feel, and sincerely caring about how I really feel inside. As a cancer patient, it is wonderful to know that a doctor or nurse is concerned about me and cares that I will get through.

Thank you for celebrating with me when I reach one year or five years in remission. I appreciate your handshake or pat on the back. Bring in the cake or the candy! Remission is an accomplishment for both of us ~ share that joy with me. Every year a cancer patient stays in remission is a gift from above. Thank you for helping to make that possible.

Thank you for taking my hand, putting your arm around me, or just giving me a hug. Whether the report is good or bad, or it's a general checkup, it is so good to share those emotions. A hug can make life easier to handle for that moment.

Thank you most of all for being my friend. As cancer patients we may have many people care about us. Sometimes a friend or spouse can't really understand our feelings because they have not been in the same situation. Thank you for understanding those feelings and fears and for being that friend who helps us get through each day.

Unless you have been a cancer patient, one cannot understand how important these "little things" are to us. Thank you to all our doctors, nurses, and technicians who take care of our needs and give of themselves to make our illness easier to cope with each and every day. Everyone of you has shown such love and given us something special in your own individual way. Keep up the good work and keep doing what you naturally do so well.

Spring 1994

You're All Done With Your Treatments-
Now What Do You Do?

by Ellen Holman

Congratulations! You're finally done with those treatments ~ either radiation, chemotherapy or a combination of both. At this point you may feel like a pin cushion, a fried egg, or a piece of meat that has been cut up and stitched a few too many times.

I know the feeling. I'm also a cancer patient who has had several surgeries plus several months of radiation. I also received nine months of chemotherapy for my type of cancer, Hodgkin's disease. It has been five years since my chemotherapy, and I am now in remission.

Cancer patients seem to express a common feeling after their treatments: "I'm so tired!" Our bodies feel as if they have been through a ringer washer with extra aches and pains that we never had before. In addition to losing our hair, we have perhaps lost weight, gained weight, lost our appetite and our sense of taste.

During our treatments, eating is not the highlight of our day. Many cancer patients are too tired to prepare a meal and perhaps too nauseous to eat it. I got so tired of people telling me to "Eat, eat, eat." Even though we don't feel like it, we know we should eat nutritionally to keep up our strength.

When I finished my chemotherapy, I made up my mind that I did not want to go through the experience again. A friend gave me a book about nutrition for good health.

Cancer is a lifetime battle that is not over and done with when your treatments are completed. You must rebuild your body after the trauma of your treatments. You are the one who must keep your body healthy by following through with good nutritional habits. Let me share with you my program that has helped to heal my body and get it on the road to recovery.

Try to include in your diet:

• Fresh fruits and vegetables. Wash all fruits and vegetables thoroughly to remove pesticides from the exterior. Steam your vegetables when cooking, but eating them raw is even better. Organic vegetables are beginning to appear on the grocery shelves, so I try to buy them when possible. Better yet, if you have space in your backyard ~ grow your own vegetables and freeze what you can for the winter. Try to avoid any canned produce.

- Meats, such as chicken, beef, veal, lamb, and fish. Venison is excellent if you have a hunter in the family. It has very little fat. Always bake or broil your meat. If you periodically do fry some meats ~ use Canola oil, but use it sparingly.

- Cooked cereals. They are so much more nutritious than dry cereals. Oatmeal, grits, cream of wheat, and buckwheat are a good variety to choose from for your breakfast. There are many multi-grain cereals but make sure they do not contain sugar.

- Eggs. Check with your doctor. As long as you exercise, eggs shouldn't hurt your cholesterol. I buy organic eggs; they taste delicious and are better for you. Avoid egg substitutes.

- Fruit and vegetable juices. These contain so many important vitamins and minerals. I love to combine carrot juice with celery juice to make a delicious vegetable drink. By blending different kinds of vegetables, you can make a great tasting vegetable juice. It does take time to make these juices, but it's well worth it because of what juices can do to help keep you well.

    Try to avoid:

- Sugar and sugar substitutes. There are so many alternative ways to sweeten foods and baked products. I use honey (sparingly), maple syrup, molasses, fruit juices, and raisins.

- White flour. Use a variety of flours such as wheat, spelt, buckwheat etc. I eat multi-grain or seven grain breads. They taste delicious and are so much better for you than just wheat or white bread.

- Preservatives. Read all package labels before buying to be sure the product contains all natural ingredients.

- Coffee and tea. There is a large variety of herbal teas that are better than plain tea. I have also bought coffee substitutes that are very close to coffee.

    Other quick points:

- Use butter instead of margarine ~ it's natural. Eat brown rice instead of white rice. Sweet potatoes are much more nutritious than white potatoes.

- Avoid cold cuts which contain nitrates. Avoid sodas ~ there is nothing nutritious in them. Health food stores contain very tasty sodas made with fruit juice. I also buy my condiments at health food stores, especially ketchup, mayonnaise, and mustard.

- Vitamins are essential. Check with your doctor before taking vitamins and also have him/her prescribe correct dosages.

Try following these guidelines. You will feel better and your body will slowly start to rebuild from your treatments.

Good luck to you and may you have a beautiful, healthy, cancer-free life.

Winter 1994

The Back Room

by Ellen Holman

In September 1986 I made my debut in the Radiation Oncology Department at Mercy Hospital in Scranton. I was 32 years old, recently divorced with two small children. My diagnosis was cancer: Hodgkin's disease, a type of lymphoma. My initial feelings could only be described in a few words: "scared to death."

As though it were yesterday, I can remember sitting in the waiting area. There were many other cancer patients sitting in that room with me. Some talked to each other, but many did not. I remember that first day as being one of the most difficult and longest days of my life. I was waiting to see the doctor to find out if I would survive the disease.

It is now five years since that day and I have returned to radiation oncology, but not for treatments. Fortunately, I am now in remission. I work as a volunteer helping other patients get through that very difficult first day, as well as those long weeks of treatment that lie ahead.

In the short time I've spent in the department I've met some very "special" cancer patients. These "special" people meet every day in what we call the *Back Room*. This is the area where they change into gowns and wait to be taken for their treatment.

This *Back Room* is colorfully decorated and has a warm, comfortable atmosphere. One of the favorite attractions is the enormous fish tank. This pleasant place is where the patients spend much of their time during the course of their treatments.

Since most patients frequent this *Back Room* each and every day, they get to know the familiar faces of other people. They become quite close. As one of them described to me, "We are like one big happy family."

As the patients get to know each other, they share their thoughts and feelings about their illness. Talking about the cancer helps to make dealing with it a little bit easier, especially when you know you're not alone. We don't spend all our time talking about cancer, we share so many other interests such as hobbies, recipes, sports, vacations, and families. Now and then someone will bring a photo of a grandchild or a special event to share with each of us.

Considering the fact that these patients were once strangers, the communication that develops over the weeks of treatment is astounding. One of the wives of a patient brought a very thick book to read while her husband was undergoing treatment. When I saw her at the end of his therapy, I asked her if she had finished her book. She told me that she had only read to page three! She explained that she had spent all her time talking and sharing with everyone else.

By the end of their treatments they all know something about each other because of all the time spent together. Some become friends and keep in touch by exchanging telephone numbers and even visiting one another at home. These people care about each other so much!

Some of the patients travel by van and come long distances. At times, a member of such a group may have to stay longer at the hospital for a specific reason. This means the other patients in the group must wait for that person before they can all go home on the van together. Not once have I heard a single complaint because of a delay. This shows how devoted they are to each other.

If one individual misses a treatment, the other patients are concerned. If they happen to have their telephone number, you can be sure that person will get a phone call later that day.

The *Back Room* people have a great sense of humor. Through all the fear, aggravation and sometimes the pain, they manage to smile and laugh. Most of the patients walk in each day with a big smile and say "Hello ~ how are you?" Many of them don't feel that well, but still manage that bright smile.

We can even joke about such things as losing hair. Leave it to a cancer patient to make hair loss an amusing topic! We share funny tales of the many experiences we've encountered in dealing with baldness and the nuisances of wearing a wig.

I don't think anyone has as much strength and endurance as these people. These soldiers encounter so many ups and downs throughout their illness. Monday tends to be the hardest day, because it means starting another week of treatments. Patients may feel weak, nauseated, or fatigued and have other side effects. Many have chemotherapy along with the radiation treatments, and also have those side effects to tolerate. Some patients have surgery before or after their treatments. A person can only handle so much, and yet these survivors keep on going. They don't want to give up, so they keep on fighting the battle. So many of them have such a very strong faith - and I know that helps them too. They encourage each other and won't let another patient give up. They are generous with reassuring words, as well as a good hug, or an arm around the shoulder. Little do these patients realize that as they care for each other they are gaining strength for themselves.

The *Back Room* is not only a special place for patients, but also a support group for the patients' spouse, children, relatives, and friends. These loved ones also share their feelings and concerns with others experiencing the same pain. Just talking about their own problems can help the loved one get through this ordeal a little easier.

Cancer is a disease that does not effect the patient alone. It touches the whole family. These survivors and their families need the support they find in the *Back Room*. Some patients do not have immediate families to give them assistance. Some older people have outlived their relatives or have no one close enough to help. For these people their only relief is found in the *Back Room.*

Some of these people have a great deal of physical pain, some have little or no support at home, and some suffer broken hearts from the loss of a loved one. These cancer patients try to put aside their fears and pain, and make the best of the situation. Some will survive their illness or at least go into remission. There are others who are grateful for the life they have had. If God grants them more time then it's a blessing. I have heard many of our older patients remark, "Life has been good to me. If it is my time to go then that's all right too."

There is an aura of love that permeates this room. You cannot see it, but each of us can feel it. There is a special closeness we experience because we are cancer survivors. Yes, we are special people because we can survive through these difficult days together. These people have given so much to me. I only hope I have been able to give as much to them.

Winter 1992

CYNTHIA HUGHES

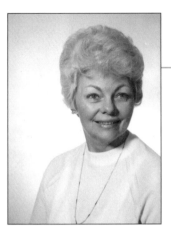

Cynthia Hughes says that almost twenty years after her first diagnosis of cancer, she always finds it wonderful to be able to look forward to holidays and special occasions. Christmas of 1995 was especially meaningful for her after her "long road back to recovery" from chemotherapy that began in 1994 for her lung cancer. A three-time survivor of cancer, Cynthia is looking forward to many more holiday celebrations.

Special Thanks!

Every Thanksgiving I say a special, personal thanks and I remember Thanksgiving Day, 1976.

My doctor was adamant about not waiting any longer for surgery on my right breast, which he had been monitoring for about six weeks. The surgeon concurred that the time had come to see what was causing the "dimpling" and "lumpiness". Since I had a history of developing benign breast cysts, it was questionable whether the manual exam was indicating a cancerous lump or just one of the many "cysty" things that were often apparent. Those were the days before mammography was used to help in breast cancer detection.

Surgery was scheduled for Friday morning, the day after Thanksgiving. I was admitted to the hospital Thursday afternoon. Neither my dear husband nor I had any appetite for a traditional holiday meal, so we went down to the hospital basement where there was a room with vending machines and we each had a cheese sandwich and a cup of coffee. It was not the least bit like Thanksgiving!

That evening I signed a paper giving my surgeon permission to remove the right breast should he deem it necessary. At that point I didn't feel very "thankful," but I tried to be cheerful in front of my husband who was visibly nervous.

When I woke up in my room, my loving sister, who is a nurse, told me that the surgery did indeed result in a modified radical mastectomy. She and the rest of my family have always been so supportive that I really never experienced the common "Why me?" attitude. The doctor gave me a reasonable amount of assurance that the surgery was successful and that no further treatment was necessary.

I recovered quickly and returned to my job as soon as possible. The only negative thought that haunted me was that I would have to wear the prosthesis every day for the rest of my life. But that was soon second nature, and the negativeness has long since passed.

Six years later, in the summer of 1982 a small lump about the size of a pea appeared directly in the middle of my mastectomy scar. After examination by my doctor, we both decided that a surgeon's opinion would be a good thing, and it was. Shortly thereafter, my second malignant lump was removed.

At the same time, a questionable lump was detected in my left breast, and a biopsy was needed for that also. When my surgeon came into my room after the biopsy, I could hear him before I could see him. He was calling out "It's benign ~ it's benign!" SWEET WORDS ! !

From then on, the seven-month follow-up treatment for the second malignant lump was thorough and intense. Bone scans, liver scans, CT-scans, chemotherapy (5FU, Methotrexate, Cytoxan, Tamoxifen), radiation therapy, hair loss, wigs, and many, many blood tests were all a part of my life. My medical and radiation oncologists had worked out a thorough master plan to defeat my cancer.

I thank God for the dedication and intelligence of the oncology professionals who worked with me. Their treatment plans were effective, and I'm proud to be a 16 year cancer survivor. We are lucky to have such able medical personnel in Northeastern Pennsylvania.

In addition to their technical skills, they also have a warm bedside manner. Their personal care and interest help create a very positive attitude, which as many of us believe, is half or maybe even three-quarters of the battle. I for one say "Thank you, doctors and nurses, for what you have done for me!"

Winter 1993

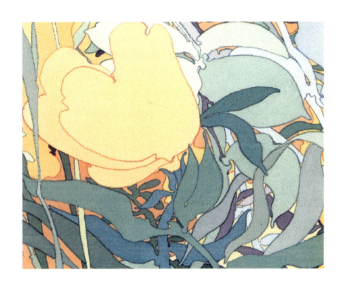

SUSAN IDE

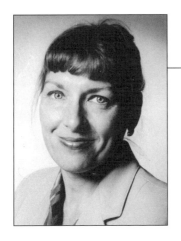

Susan Ide, former Associate Professor of English at Keystone College, died in November 1993, three years after her diagnosis of breast cancer. Her friends and colleagues are establishing a memorial garden at Keystone to honor Susan and her special contributions to her students.

Lump

"The lump~
Amorphous and amoral~
Is an archetype of magic,"
lectured the anthropologist.
"Shape it, name it,
Kiss it with breath:
It leaps to life.
Shape it, name it,
Stab it with pins:
Someone dies."

Mountains
Are an archetype of mother.
The Appalachians nudge
Out of morning mists
Like the breasts of a woman
Sleeping in a gauzy nightgown.
I can almost see her breathe.
I want to press my head in the hollow.

I want the soft mountain breasts to stop my ears,
The veil to block my eyes,
The mammoth strength of mountains
To protect and comfort me.
The lump in my breast
Has no shape or name.
All day I kick it ahead of me
Like a sidewalk stone.
I try to control the magic,
Avoiding cracks, wishing on dandelions.
But I am afraid.

There's a macrocosmic magic
Beyond star wishes
Where happiness is taboo.
Now I want to live 3,000 years
To love him,
Death incubates in my breast.

My Seventeen Year Old Daughter and I Pick Blueberries

by Susan Ide

We kneel among myriad green mandalas,
Palming hosts of blueberries.
We keep silent.
We listen for slithering,
Since snakes hide in blueberries.
We are gathering ourselves.
Each berry a woman's breast;
Each blue globe a world
Like earth viewed from the moon.
We are Earth Mothers and
Daughters of Earth.
We keep silent.
We Hear Eve breathe in Eden.

Spring 1995

Sumac with Robins

by Susan Ide

At two thousand feet in March in Pennsylvania
A flock of robins makes a dawn landing:
A hundred ravenous robins and one staghorn sumac
With perches for thirty-three at a time.
Rusty red breasts brush rusty red clusters.
Empty robins wait in the dead oak on the right,
The replete wait in the dead oak on the left.
Who is the happiest?
The robins anticipating sumac?
The robins gorging on the breast-red berries?
The striped staghorn at noon that fed them?
The conscious, observing eye?

Love Knot

by Susan Ide

The love knot as a symble for infinity
Was the brainchild of John Wallis,
Renaissance mathematician in England,
Where, since ancient times, folks sang
Of holly and ivy and shaped them into
Leafy wreaths to celebrate love's embrace.
Emblem of all Christmas commemorates:
The Grace, the Mystery, the Limitless.
And here I wish you these infinitives:
To love, to laugh, to learn, to wonder, and to praise.

Laundry on a Line

by Susan Ide

Laundry on a line
Transports her.
Striped shirts and skirts
Stretch and puff like spinnakers;
White sheets pregnant with wind
Move her like mainsails.
Her fingers, calloused and water-ridged,
Handle with sailors facility
Rope, pully, and worn wet wood.
Her eye is sharp to weather,
Discriminating shades of blue
In sky boundless as ocean.
Sun tans and toughens her skin like love.
Moist scent of honeysuckle
Hints unseen islands.
Dreams are clean here.
Power is private.
Obedient to physical laws,
She is master of the ship.

Privileges of the Doomed

by Susan Ide

To lie long in bed listening to birdsong,
To stand long looking at dandelions,
To eat chocolate,
To tell the truth,
To hug and kiss
Everyone.

CASSIE KOBESKI

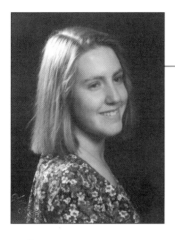

Cassie Kobeski, who was 13 when she wrote this essay, is now a 16 year old junior at Dunmore High School, where she enjoys writing and art. She is thankful for the important lessons she learned from her aunt's diagnosis of cancer, and that her aunt remains a healthy survivor.

"Imagine That"...Imagining Life Without Her

When I think about it, my day was going all right. It was an average day; everything seemed normal until my mother came upstairs. We were going to the mall; it was a weekday, around 6:00 pm. I was trying to fix my hair.

My aunt, around two days earlier went for a mammogram. The results came back that day and my mother said to me "Remember when Aunt Ranny went for that mammogram? Well the results came back and they found a lump."

"Could it be cancer?" ... I was familiar with the subject because my grandmother had breast cancer some years ago.

"Yes," my mother answered.

At that I started to break into tears. My mother must have already cried because her eyes were all red and puffy but she joined in with me anyway.

We went to the mall and anything would make me cry. No matter if it was a song, a picture, or a word.

You never realize how much someone or something means to you until someone or something threatens to take them away from you. When you imagine life without the people you love and care about it seems so empty. I experienced many deaths in my family and I didn't want to experience another one. Especially my Aunt Ranny, who I am very close to. She is like a second mother to me but also a friend. She is one of the most beautiful, wonderful, strong, intelligent, caring, and loving people I have ever met. She is a person who I love, respect, and trust unconditionally for her strength and courage through all this.

I am not writing this to win a prize. I am writing this to express my feeling in imagining life without my aunt. It wouldn't be right. I know now not to take people or things you love or cherish for granted. Sometimes it's too late and you don't get a chance to say good-bye to them. But luckily in my case my aunt is still living. She had a breast removed and today is taking chemotherapy. But what is that compared to the most precious gift of life? I think the thing that helped her most through all this is the love and support from her family and friends.

When I get older I hope to find a cure for cancer and I will dedicate it to all the people who have died from cancer, fought it, or lost a loved one from it.

Winter 1993

CONNIE LASHEVICKI

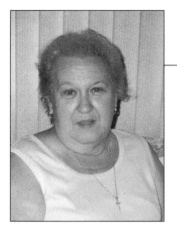

Connie Lashevicki enjoys her retirement and the chance to savor life with her husband of 39 years, Stanley, and their three daughters and four grandchildren. She continues to encourage women to take personal responsibility for their health, especially through regular mammography, breast self examination, and physician exams.

One Hour A Year Can Save Your Life

I am writing this article as my 5 year anniversary of surviving breast cancer has just passed. I wish I could get this message across to all women to make sure they have a mammogram every year with their yearly checkup.

My experience with breast cancer was very scary. I never had a mammogram until I was 55 years old. The doctor I went to then never suggested having one. Well, when he moved out of our town, I started going to a new doctor who eventually saved my life. As a new patient, I had to have a complete checkup and a mammogram. A few days after my mammogram, my doctor called and said "something showed up" on it. On June 29, 1990, I had a biopsy. It seemed like a lifetime while waiting for

the results. The surgeon called on July 3rd and told me that the lump in my breast was cancerous. One week after my biopsy, on July 6th, the lump, which was the size of a pea, was removed along with eight lymph nodes.

After my operation, my family doctor set up an appointment with a medical oncologist and a radiation oncologist. Under their care I received 25 radiation treatments.

A year and a half later, at my yearly checkup, "something showed up" again on my mammogram. My family doctor wanted me to see a surgeon, but the fear of going through another operation really upset me. I called my oncologist and explained my concerns about having another biopsy, so he set up a Mammotest. This procedure was fairly new at the time and I was one of the first to have it done. Fortunately, this time the results showed no cancer.

The word cancer is not new to me. In 1957, I was married only 9 months when my 49 year old mother-in-law died of ovarian cancer; my mom died of colon cancer in 1981; and just recently in February 1995 my son-in-law, who was just 35 years old, died of lung cancer.

No one likes to hear that they have cancer, but remember if it is found in time you can be helped. My lump was the size of a pea. The doctors said that if I had not had the mammogram that detected the problem, I would not have been able to feel the lump for another year, and by that time it might have been too late to assume I would have been a survivor.

After surviving cancer for 5 years, I thank the Lord for the help of my doctors, family and friends.

I am taking the drug Tamoxifen to help guard against a recurrence of breast cancer and still go to the doctor for regular check ups.

I hope this article will get my message across: remember to stress to your friends, your family members, and yourself to have a yearly mammogram.

Fall 1995

NANCY LEACH

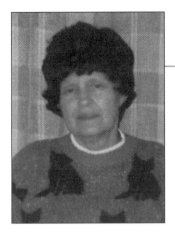

Nancy Leach discovered that poetry was the best way for her to express her deep religious faith. Her husband Allen included 82 of her poems in a book entitled "All Sufficient Grace" which he published only a few months after Nancy died from cancer in February 1994. Nancy wrote this poem while undergoing chemotherapy shortly after her diagnosis of malignant myeloma in 1992.

"Cancer"

Challenged from without,
within this cancer verdict, can it win?
Bodies aching, racked with pain,
cancer is it's very name.

From without there is much doubt,
How can I live and see this out?
I am frail and weak you see
Why did this happen now to me?

Let me look, for now I know
This challenge is for me to show,
All my strength and inner beauty
For to man this is my duty.

Then God will I be true
As in his power I give to you.
All the hope and joy of knowing
Healing, life is ever growing.

Challenge met and victory won
Only God can overcome,
Fear and anguish fade away
As we live another day.

Spring 1993

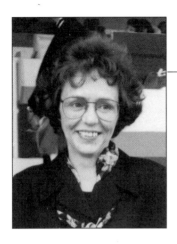

JANE LININGER

Jane Lininger, a.k.a., Happy Thawts is still on-line and doing well! Not only does she enjoy "chatting" with her friends on-line but she also is actively involved in the "Facing Cancer Together" support group at Mercy Hospital Cancer Center. She enjoys spending time with her three children Melissa, T.J., and Patrick.

Happy Thawts

In January 1994, I was diagnosed with pancreatic cancer. During my recovery after surgery, chemotherapy and radiation therapy, I tried to think of my illness as a long-term cold. With determination, defiance, a great support system, and a lot of spunk, I knew I would overcome this cruel interruption in my life. My main focus was my children and my work. I believed returning to work would mean I was well, and all my troubles would be behind me.

In August 1994 I did, indeed, return to work. Shortly afterward, like being struck by lightening, I realized I wanted to *live*, not exist in a rat race of working and raising a family. By January 1995 I was no longer employed. Faced with my voluntary retirement, I had to decide what to do with all the time on my hands.

With the help of a few computer-literate friends, I purchased a computer, complete with software for on-line services. I had no computer training, and I felt that my children would benefit most. Well, guess what? Now they have to fight me for their computer time!

America On-line, my software package, is one of several telecommunication on-line services. A valuable resource of almost infinite potential, it is a community of people from all across America, a vast network of members. People meeting people, friends chatting with friends, family members catching up with one another. The 90's way to communicate!

Anyone with a computer, a telephone line, and familiarity with a typewriter keyboard can join the on-line "conversations". In only a few weeks I became comfortable moving through the computer world, and I discovered Health Forum, a network of health-related information posted on computer message boards. Just recently, the American Cancer Society joined the forum.

I found there was quite a variety of messages on the forum asking for cancer information or offering support to fellow cancer patients. I posted a message requesting anyone with information on pancreatic cancer to contact me. The response was wonderful! I now correspond regularly with two fellow members: one a pancreatic cancer patient and one a physician's assistant whose father was recently diagnosed with pancreatic cancer.

Also included in the forum are weekly support groups that meet on-line. These are live conversations, typed by the participants on their keyboard, that appear on screen. There are two "hosts" who greet each new person in the group. Some are well-informed lay people, while others are trained professionals willing to help anyone seeking information or to lend a compassionate ear. "Listening" to conversations on a computer screen may seem cold and impersonal, but you can actually feel the pain of another group member going through treatment. The agony and uncertainty of recent diagnosis, the joy of remission, and the fear of pending tests. These sessions can provide a wealth of information or welcome comfort when you most need it.

Anonymity allows many to express thoughts or feelings that perhaps wouldn't come easily in a personal meeting. You may sit and watch conversations roll by, without comment, or you may feel compelled to respond. Either is acceptable. The more people in the group, the faster the words roll by. I have seen as few as 26 people in the forum and as many as 40 people participating in the conversation.

Support groups on-line are not a substitute for an actual support meeting, but can be a wonderful supplemental gathering, the privilege of personal contact and conversation without leaving home. Without my family, my friends, and my real support group, "Facing Cancer Together" at the Mercy Hospital Cancer Center in Scranton, I am certain I would not be where I am today. I owe all of them my heartfelt thanks.

This is *Happy Thawts* signing off and inviting you all to join us on-line!

Summer 1995

JOHN A. McCOLE

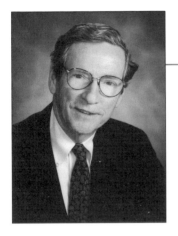

John McCole is remembered by his myriad of friends as a man whose character was woven with a rare fabric of durability and grace ~ a combination of tough anthracite courage and loyalty, guilded by warm and infectious charm. His irrepressible love of life and perpetual optimism were an inspiration to all, and he was quick to share his message of hope and encouragement with other people living with cancer. John, who was a speaker at NRCI's 1993 *Survivors Celebration*, died in September 1994.

Can This Be Happening to Me?

Shock! Disbelief! Shock!

These were my first reactions when I heard my diagnosis of lymphoma cancer with bone involvement.

Why me? No one in my family had cancer. I was a runner for many years, had watched my eating and dietary habits, and did all I could to stay in good health. Yet, my diagnosis was confirmed by numerous tests.

I had been experiencing some medical difficulties, but early studies indicated only minor problems similar to a viral infection. Fortunately, my physician encouraged me to undergo further testing, and these provided the concrete diagnosis of lymphoma. This meant the disease was throughout my lymphatic system.

After the initial shock began to subside, I was able to listen and respond to the thoughtful and helpful words of many concerned friends. Their phone calls, letters, books, tapes, and even prayers contributed to my realization of how important a positive attitude can be, and also that my personal, psychological acceptance of my cancer diagnosis could give me the best chance for a recovery, cure, or remission.

As a matter of fact, the kindness of so many people made it almost ~ but not quite! ~ worth having to deal with the disease.

Medically, I've had great support from a team of physicians and oncology specialists. In addition, the nursing staff in my oncologist's office as well as at two local hospitals have been very caring. In general, friends have continued to go beyond the call of duty by visiting, keeping in touch through cards and letters, as well as by giving me books and tapes about coping with cancer.

I am particularly grateful for the concern and care of my spouse and the rest of my family, who all have been very supportive. It is often difficult for families, particularly when treatment frequently leaves the patient in a state of agitation. I hope further studies of these psychological difficulties and reactions to cancer treatment will yield benefits for the patient, family, and friends.

It was a surprise to me to learn that 1 out of 3 people in America will develop cancer. These alarming statistics are magnified, because a cancer diagnosis also affects other family members. Cancer strikes 3 out of 4 families. I was totally unaware of this reality until I was personally touched by the disease.

Certainly, one needs a positive attitude in order to cope with any life threatening illness and, hopefully, to recover. For many people, this means a change in priorities, personal adjustments, and an inventory of values. Believe me, good medicine is vital; yet equally important is family support and the support of friends, including fellow cancer patients.

For many people an ability to keep a normal work schedule, though at times difficult, has therapeutic benefits. I was able to get out every day, even though some days required a shorter schedule and a slower pace.

Naturally the weekly visits to the doctor and the various treatments make a normal work routine difficult. Yet my recommendation would be that if health permits, keeping busy with your daily occupation is a very good prescription for an improved mental attitude, which can help recovery. My colleagues at MONY/Mutual of New York offered wonderful support and encouragement.

It also can be enormously helpful to talk with friends whose families have experienced the diagnosis and treatment of cancer, and with other wonderful people who have special empathy for those afflicted. People who come forward to guide and support cancer patients are indeed a major plus in the fight. I think this personal interplay among those touched by the disease is unique.

As mentioned, a positive attitude is important for your recovery and well-being. For example, the Bernie Siegel tapes have great therapeutic value. They can really help you understand and experience the mind-body connection and teach you to focus on positive thoughts. In fact, I think, if you are not positive in your outlook, you may well find yourself fighting your disease alone. You cannot expect continual support from your friends and your associates if your attitude is continually negative.

Finally, though it may seem like an old or trite refrain, prayers from your friends, your family, and you personally are still one of today's strongest medicines.

Winter 1993

REVEREND BILL NELSON

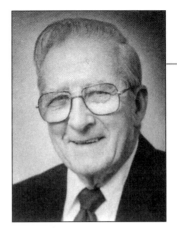

Bill Nelson says that "like the Energizer Bunny, I just go on, and on, and on". Eight years after his cancer treatment, Reverend Nelson still finds that keeping busy by helping others can, indeed, be life's best medicine. He continues to serve as pastor for Beaver Meadows Church in Wyoming County.

What's It Like?

What's it like? That's the question people ask most. They are not prying. They are not impolite. They just don't understand what it is like to experience cancer. So, when they ask me I tell them what it's like.

What's the treatment like? For me, it meant radiation therapy. My first radiation treatment was a memorable experience! My doctor had explained very carefully what my course of treatment would be like, but it's difficult to be prepared for the "real thing." I walked apprehensively toward the treatment table, and climbed on with the helping hand of the technologist. As I lay down, the gantry supporting the imposing machinery loomed large above me.

The technologists reassuringly explained again what would happen. But it was ominously silent when they left me alone in the room for the actual delivery of the radiation. However, their calm, pleasant voices coming through the intercom guided me through the short, momentary treatment.

The gantry rotated. I felt nothing. The technologists returned. As they assisted me off the table, one asked "That wasn't so bad, was it?"

"Not bad at all!" I said with relief. "It gets easier each time." they said. Words of assurance. They were right.

What's it like coping with your normal daily routine during treatment? I know that depending on the particular site being treated, some patients experience problems while undergoing radiation which can interfere with their usual life style. I never did.

For me, keeping busy by helping others was the best medicine. At the time of my treatment, I was helping with a summer migrant worker program through our church in Clarks Summit. When I drove into Scranton for my daily radiation therapy at Mercy Hospital, I brought migrant workers with me for their medical appointments with other doctors at the hospital.

As soon as I finished my treatment, I picked up my passengers, returned them to our office or to their camp, and then completed my desk work for the rest of the day. Sometimes, I was a bit more tired than usual, but I never felt sick during my seven weeks of therapy.

What's it like dealing with the stress that so often accompanies cancer treatments? I found it most helpful to learn all I could about how I could help the healing process. I read everything I could get my hands on. I wanted to learn! Talking with the psychological, social, or pastoral care workers at the hospital was extremely beneficial. To this day, four and one half years after treatment, I consider learning about how to deal with stress the most valuable lesson of my experience with cancer.

Why? Well it's important that we maintain balance in all organs and functions of the body ~ a process known as homeostasis. I remember that from my college physiology course many, many years ago. What I learned during my treatment for cancer is that the experience can cause additional pressures in our already stressful lives.

Some stress can be positive. We witnessed that recently in the Winter Olympics. Under stress, our blood runs faster, our hearts pound, our muscles tense for action. That's what motivates Olympic champions. However, those same positive physical responses can be negative for those whose bodies are reacting to an outside situation ~ such as the stress of coping with disease.

Some of us become good at putting up a good front. But inside, our systems can take just so much before they are thrown out of balance. Radiation or chemotherapy may knock us out of balance psychologically and physically, making it harder to deal with the disease.

Reading books by other cancer patients and working with health care professionals helped me keep things in perspective. It actually helped restore my faith and belief in myself. Opening the door to faith is like opening doors to the rooms of a house. You open and enter one at a time. You open the door to faith in yourself, in your physician, in your treatment. You open the way to return to balance in your life.

And then, you work with others to help them through their troubles. What I learned is that helping others can, indeed, be the best medicine!

Spring 1992

Don't Bury Me Yet!

by Reverend Bill Nelson

I stepped out of the car at the funeral home. Suddenly, there was Harriet in front of me. I had come to perform the funeral of her friend.

"Oh! Reverend Bill, I heard! I heard! It's too bad!" Almost before I could think, the words burst out. . . "Don't bury me yet!"

It shook me more to hear her reaction to the news, than when I first learned I had cancer and that I needed to start radiation therapy the next Monday.

I had gone in the week before for a biopsy. John, the man in the bed next to me, had the same surgery. His daughters were so pessimistic, so down, it bothered me. I talked about it that day with John. His attitude was that he did not believe he would make it. I determined I would not go into surgery feeling like that.

When I awoke in recovery, there was the nurse. I had officiated at her wedding, had done their family taxes in my accounting service. My first words were, "You? I must be in heaven to find such a beautiful nurse." Diane chuckled. She knew me as up-beat and a tease.

Getting in the three-armed gown for my first radiation was not easy. I thought they were made for right-handers, which I am not. As I sat down, waiting my turn, the chill on my bottom made me wonder how much of me others saw that they shouldn't. The magazine I looked at was not as fascinating as the looks on the faces of those waiting. A few half smiled. Most looked very grim. I determined then that I would be up-beat, optimistic, on top, instead of pulled down by circumstances, or by people. Also, if my faith and my prayers were to work, I had to get in line with what I believed and prayed. I had to get my act together.

I'm very enthusiastic about the stress therapy program at Mercy Hospital. Having earned three degrees in guidance and counseling, I was both pleased and helped by the six hours given by the social case worker. It brought back memories of instruction and practice I had received in clinical training at Boston City Hospital, and at the Brockton Veterans Hospital.

I discovered that many do not receive stress therapy during their cancer treatment. In my mind, this initiates the healing process. As one assimilates knowledge about stress management, he or she develops attitudes that are favorable to the healing process.

Our minds, our souls, our spirits, are like sponges. Whatever we put there is absorbed. Bad thoughts, despair, anger, frustration, and stress tie our emotions in knots. Give yourself good thoughts, and you feel better. You reap what you sow. You get what you give. Stress management is important for all of life, especially when dealing with a difficult disease.

What am I doing four years after radiation? Retired three times, I'm now working three jobs because my wife is so expensive! At 70, I am Pastor at Beaver Meadows Church, work 40 hours a week in security at Taylor Beef; and have Allied Associated, where I just took on a partner to help with the workload of accounting and taxes.

Last Sunday I overheard a woman say, "I don't know where he gets the energy," I yelled back, "It ain't Geritol!"

Sunday afternoons from 4:00 to 5:30, I teach my church youngsters clowning. I love it! Been at clowning six years! My wife says, "You don't need a clown suit!" She has known me for 49 years.

Winter 1992

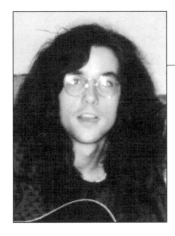

WILLIAM NORMENT

William Norment is living in North Carolina where he continues to enjoy life and to follow his philosophy: *Carpe Diem ~ Seize the Day!*

Carpe Diem!

Seminoma of the right testicle. What a shock! After the devastating impact of my diagnosis subsided I was overwhelmed by the love and concern expressed by co-workers, friends, and most importantly family. They let me know I was not alone and that I could count on them at all times. I didn't realize how much I meant to them and how much they really mean to me.

My physician and everyone at the hospital were fantastic! They soothed my fears about radiation therapy and filled in the "gaps" in my knowledge about my disease. My doctor told me how common testicular tumors are and explained the details of treatment.

I had a hard time at first, dealing with fears and being optimistic about treatment. Even though I was repeatedly told the prognosis was good, I occasionally worked myself up into an emotional frenzy. That's when family plays an important role in allaying fears and bringing back confidence. Thank heavens for family!

I was also very lucky that my wife had made me go to the doctor in the first place. I was in the habit of ignoring problems because I felt good at the time. (I have talked to other cancer patients, especially the men, and find I was not alone.) Early detection is so important! Ignoring problems has never solved them and yet we sometimes wait until it's too late.

Carpe Diem ~ Seize The Day ~ has never

meant so much to me as it does now. I catch myself smiling more and I feel good! Even the clickety-clackety sound from my old car is a sweet symphony. Positive thoughts have a great therapeutic value and are a great asset in fighting disease and despair. It sometimes takes a disaster to make us appreciate life and everyone around us.

I hope when reading this you can feel the hope and joy I so deeply have. Oh, I occasionally get sad but it's never as bad as it used to be and it never lasts long.

Could it be that I owe a debt of thanks to my disease for reminding me of the truly important things in life? Thank you!

Spring 1993

FATHER J.A. PANUSKA

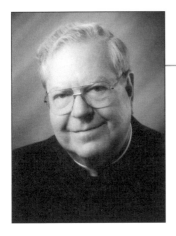

Father J. A. Panuska, SJ, a Baltimorean by birth, scientist by special academic training, Jesuit priest and educator by vocation, seeks to work in areas which generate a synergistic multiplier effect in service to others. He is most grateful that early diagnosis and curative action have allowed him to continue his work serving others. Father Panuska has been President of the University of Scranton since 1982.

Medical Detectives

I am writing this reflection during a vacation on the beach at Atlantic City. The ocean always relaxes me, and allows me to see things more clearly than when I am engulfed in the complications of life at the University.

During every vacation I try to do some light reading that most often includes mystery stories. I usually read while sitting in a beach chair under a sun-protecting umbrella, listening to the surf beat against the shore arriving near my feet in an unpredictable pattern. This takes me away from thinking about the challenges that fill my life back in Scranton.

My fondness for mystery stories reflects in a way

my many years of scientific research at St. Louis, Emory, Cambridge, and Georgetown universities. Trying to find meaning within a maze of possibly-related details is one of my pleasures. This analytic activity relates to my recent bout with cancer, and the remarkable medical detectives in Scranton whose interpretation of subtle clues resulted in my current good health.

It was early fall, and I was entering my ninth year as president at the University of Scranton, when some abnormal urinary activity provoked a visit to my family physician. At that time there seemed to be only a possible urinary infection and no specific problem with my prostate gland. The infection was promptly treated, and most of the original symptoms disappeared.

The good medical detective, however, ordered another series of blood tests just to make sure that the story was complete and that all of the evidence was in. The tests revealed that the prostate-specific antigen (PSA) that was very high at the beginning of the infection remained high even after the infection was gone.

This indicator was sufficient evidence to encourage a referral to a urologist. Several tests were undertaken, but no clear abnormalities appeared. Since, however, the PSA remained high, the urologist wisely recommended biopsies, and I readily agreed. Frankly, I expected a negative result.

A few days later, on the morning of a President's Circle Dinner at the University while I was having brunch with my family in the Jesuit Community, a phone call informed me that there was a problem: a relatively low level adenocarcinoma was found. The cells were well-differentiated, a good sign; but it was multi-focal, a bad sign. Clearly, further evaluation and probably corrective action would have to be taken.

A series of most helpful consultations followed and, as a scientist, I carefully reviewed my own pathology from both books and scientific articles, some of which were borrowed from one of my doctors. I even did a computer search on the publications of one of the consultants, and read a number of his scientific articles relating to problems like mine. The detective in me was showing through.

When finally I was told that surgery, a radical prostatectomy, was my best course, I readily assented. When I heard that my chances were good, I thought, only good? What if we were a bit late? I was told that until the surgery no definitive answer could be given.

Indeed, depending upon what was found in the lymph nodes, if anything, the surgery might not even be completed. This ran counter to my own personal desire for clear, prompt answers, but the medical detective was being honest with me. I felt a foreboding that the result would be bad. Nevertheless, despite being somewhat emotionally exhausted, I was at peace.

During the surgery an epidural anesthesia was used and, in a fuzzy way, I thought that I heard the technician tell the surgeon that the lymph nodes were clear. I remembered saying out loud. "Thank God." I later learned from my primary urologist who was present during the surgery that I had said that. Indeed, I had been quite voluble during the procedure, seeming to give directions. I guess CEO's remain CEO's even under anesthesia.

As it turned out, I required no follow-up therapy, and I was told that if I ever got cancer it would be unrelated to this particular case.

My physical recovery followed a normal pattern, and now, as I enter my eleventh year at the University of Scranton, I am in excellent physical condition with no hint of that troublesome PSA that stimulated so much activity earlier.

My experience was more than physical. There was also, although somewhat mysteriously delayed, a psychological effect. It made me more aware than ever of both the fragility and resilience of human life. I became more determined than ever to use what might indeed be many years ahead of me to be even more bold in my efforts to do good for people in my life, to intensify meaning.

The irregular patterns of the waves at the sea shore, and the repetitive sound of the surf, are akin to many events within the environment of our lives, certainly for me. Within our lives we must find a true centering point and pursue it whether we be in our twenties, forties, sixties, or beyond. We all realize this at one time or another, and an experience like mine, which I know has been shared by many, reinforces that perception.

And I for one will always be grateful to the medical detectives who solved my mystery. They found meaning in a confusing pattern of facts and pursued it to a solution; a happy conclusion which left the recipient satisfied, whole, and more purposeful.

Fall 1992

JACK RACE

Jack Race has dedicated his life to his personal ethic: Love all people everywhere, reaching out in kindness, compassion, and service. After more than thirty years as a pilot with PanAm, Jack served as a volunteer for eight years as Chief Pilot for Project Orbis to help combat blindness throughout the world. He also helps counsel men who are dealing with their diagnosis and treatment of prostate cancer and is a lay pastor with the American Baptist Church.

Two Are Better Than One

In the story "The Little Prince" by Antoine DeSaint Exupery there is a line that is a very simple yet almost secret truth:

"It is only with the heart that one can see rightly; what is essential is invisible to the eye."

As a cancer survivor this simple truth has been an important part of my life.

What is essential is to look out on our wounded world with a heart of love. See if there is some little thing we can do for another ~ some kindness, some compassion, some service. Something we can do here and there and now and then.

Of course there will be failures ~ at least there have been for me. But I'm taken away from the "Why me?" and the many other inward turning thoughts we are subject to in illness.

Even though cancer is still a part of my life I somehow have experienced a kind of fulfillment these recent years, and yet in this experience I know I cannot stand alone. I need others ~ as we all do.

There is a splendid passage from the Bible which speaks to this truth, from Ecclesiastes these words:

"Two are better than one... if one falls down his friend can help him up. But pity the person who falls and has no one to help him up! ...a cord of three strands is not quickly broken."

What a marvelous truth in these words!

As I accept this and understand that what is

essential in life is seen best with the heart, then a center outside one's self can be created and we can help one another up.

For cancer survivors ~ as well as for everyone ~ I think we need to love ourselves, i.e. to know we are of value and have something to offer this world. Only in this can we have hope. And to have joy in our lives we need to know that another loves and cares about us.

Fulfillment comes through reaching out and loving others.

Winter 1995

KAREN RUMENSKY

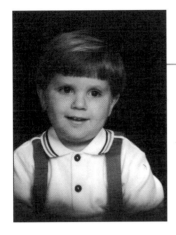

Karen Rumensky and her family continue to be inspired by their son Michael's spirited strength and courage after the innumerable medical complications he endured before, during, and after his bone marrow transplant procedure. At their first opportunity to meet one year post-transplant, three year old Michael and his bone marrow donor Jay Davis developed a uniquely spontaneous personal bond, and the beauty of their special love is shared by the entire Rumensky family.

Gifts From a Child and a Stranger

Life

It's supposed to be so easy. A couple enters into marriage, decides to have children, and through love and dedication a wonderful family is born. As we grow and progress, each family member is able to draw strength from the other. For our family, this strength is drawn from the courage of our three year old son.

Diagnosis

After a routine checkup in April 1993, our 1 year old son Michael was diagnosed with pre-leukemia. After repeated visits to many specialists, Michael was diagnosed with Juvenile Chronic Myelogenous Leukemia (JCML), a rare form of leukemia uncommon for children

Michael's age.

For us, it was as if the doctors had delivered his death sentence. Our days consisted of trips to the hospital for blood work and our constant prayers for miracles. Standard chemotherapy is not effective for this type of cancer and Michael's only chance for survival was a bone marrow transplant. No one in our immediate family was a suitable match to donate marrow for Michael, so we registered him with the National Bone Marrow Donor Program (NBMDP). The doctors said chances for a perfect match were slim.

We were overwhelmed by the new language and terms used by his doctors, and decided to learn as much as possible about his disease. We contacted the American

Cancer Society, Leukemia Society, National Cancer Institute, and the Candlelighters Foundation and they gave us books and information we could understand. We learned that each and every cancer patient is different, and that Michael was not your typical text book case.

Hope and Healing Begin

Children's Hospital of Philadelphia (CHOP) notified us in November 1993 that a full match bone marrow donor had been located, and Michael could begin what we hoped would be the healing process. Michael underwent surgery to prepare him for the bone marrow transplant and to remove his enlarged spleen. We returned home to Dickson City to celebrate a "normal" Christmas. Our Christmas was all but normal. Michael quickly became ill and his transplant accelerated. Two days after Christmas we headed to CHOP for Michael's extensive chemotherapy and total body radiation to destroy his diseased bone marrow. On January 6, 1994, he received a matched unrelated donors (MUD) bone marrow.

The Waiting Game

After Michael's bone marrow transplant, we began a waiting game for the marrow to engraft in Michael's body. We watched our perky little boy get sicker and sicker. We look back now and understand that to help him get better we had to make him sick. Slowly, the dark days began to look brighter as we saw a bounce in Michael as he courageously began fighting back.

Michael was discharged 27 days after transplant, but he had a long fight as his severely compromised immune system was challenged by many infections. He suffered numerous physical setbacks in the next nine months as he and we suffered through his body's attempts to accept the new marrow, bouts with tube feedings, a respiratory problem after exposure to chicken pox, and kidney failure. Kidney medication caused stress on Michael's heart muscles, resulting in his re-admission to CHOP with chronic heart failure.

The Strength of a Child

Since undergoing surgery, chemotherapy, radiation, a bone marrow transplant, and numerous infections and treatments, Michael seems to have resumed his "normal" life as a three year old. Perhaps the main reason for Michael's spirited rebound stems from the fact that he is a child and simply does not realize the severity of the situation. We have all been able to draw strength from his courage. Michael's resilience is wonderful. He is the reason we keep going each day. When we look at him and he smiles back, we know we made the right choice. In January 1995, one year post transplant for Michael, we received wonderful reports from his doctors that he was recovering well.

The Mysterious Donor

One year before Michael's good report, a mysterious donor decided to give up his Christmas vacation in order to aid our son. We pledged that no matter what happened to Michael, we would meet this tremendous person who gave the hope of life to our son. Restrictions of the NBMDP stipulate that the donor and the recipient may not meet until one year after transplant. Our donor was, however, allowed to contact Michael via an anonymous letter. This letter is reprinted with our story.

One year after the transplant we had the wonderful opportunity to meet Michael's donor, Jay. We consider Jay as Michael's guardian angel who gave us the greatest gift: a second chance for life, and 18 months of joy with our vibrant 3 year old son.

After meeting Jay, we learned of the tragic circumstances that made our miracle possible. In 1989 a professor at Dartmouth College was diagnosed with leukemia, and Jay was one of the hundreds of students who volunteered to be tested for a possible match. Though he did not know the professor, Jay had heard wonderful things about him, and was truly disappointed when no suitable match could be found to save his life.

The professor's reputation and compassion for his students did, however, save our son Michael. Because Jay had been tested in an attempt to save the professor's life, he was entered into the NBMDP. In Jay's words, "Michael is a very healthy child. Michael is something very positive that has come out of the tragedy of the professor's struggle with his disease."

We will be forever grateful to Jay. He and his wife Julie have become a wonderful part of our lives, thoughts and prayers.

A New Life

Every day Michael sings the Disney song "It's a Small World" and every night Michael remembers Jay, Julie, and Jay's kitty cat Jasmine in his prayers. When we listen to our childrens' prayers, their prayers for each other, and for hope and cures for the children of tomorrow, we realize they are our link to the future. To look at Michael, he is the picture of health who is full of life and love, and we are grateful to Jay for our little miracle, a stranger who became our friend.

Our hope for other parents is that each day they appreciate their children's gentle smiles and hugs, as they watch them play and sing songs and see the twinkle and magic inside them. We say to them never give up; keep your faith and your appreciation and your love for your family and friends. Life is a precious gift.

Dear Recipient of My Marrow,

I am writing this the night before my (our) operation, with the knowledge that in around ten hours they are going to be taking something out of me that might save your life. This is a staggeringly powerful and sobering thought for me ~ that you might be able to lead a more normal life because of a little bit of fluid that is sitting in my bones right now. People have wished me well today, telling me how impressed they are by the "sacrifice" I am making tomorrow. I know, however, that this "sacrifice" is nothing compared to the sacrifices, emotional and physical, that you and your parents have been making every day for the last year. I do not know your family but I know you must all have incredible courage and faith and love for each other. I am incredibly lucky to have led a healthy life to this point, and I only hope that the health I have been given will somehow transfer into your little body, allowing it to continue its wonderful struggle to live and grow old. I do not know if our operations tomorrow will work and I do not like even admitting the possibility that they might not. I want you to know, though, that I have put a lot of positive, healthy thoughts into my bones over the last two months, and these thoughts will stay in my marrow when it becomes your marrow. I wish you a wonderful life.

Your Bone Marrow Donor

Summer 1995

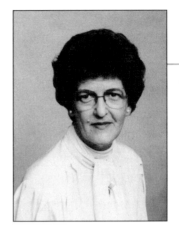

JOYCE SCHWINN

Joyce Schwinn is remembered fondly as a teacher, musician, writer, and lover of the arts; a lady who challenged not only her students, but also herself. Diagnosed with cancer in the spring of 1991, she died in the fall of 1994 after a courageous struggle through chemotherapy, radiation therapy, and surgery. Those who knew Joyce know that she continues to live in the hearts and minds of the many people of all ages whom she touched, encouraged, and inspired.

You Can Make a Difference

In remission. Magical words! When I asked one of my doctors to be specific about its meaning in terms of recurrence, I kept hearing YOU.

"You responded well to treatment." "You tolerated the radiation well." "If this continues, you..."

The operative word, it seemed, was *you* and *your*, meaning me and mine. So I'll claim my cancer and my remission and pursue the meaning of *you* in all this, if you will allow me.

It would be easy and simplistic to offer my generic solutions as a cure-all. That's not how it works. *You* truly is the operative word. There are as many different cancers as there are people who get the disease. And the variety of treatments, thank God, are in the talented

minds and gentle hands of the technologists, nurses, and doctors who work in all the phases of oncology. The patient, however, plays a very, very important part in the outcome of that treatment and the *you* within you can make an immense difference.

Cope, if and when you can, with humor. Yes, humor! I was born, I think, with an abundant sense of it that has been fostered throughout my life by family, friends, and colleagues. It serves me well.

Try it! When all the equipment gets attached for chemotherapy and you're still mobile, you might as well walk around playing the strolling robot. When the wheels on the pole want to go north and south at the same time, the tubing gets snarled in the coffee machine, and the whole damn thing starts lurching at you and your poor overworked nurse, throw up your hands, call it names, cuss a bit, and get on with it.

Be grateful, if you can, that you feel well enough to get annoyed, if not downright angry. Furious can be funny. Just don't try it on your nurses; they're your lifeline in calmer moments.

When the orderlies and various attendants and helpers come to cart you off for one more annoying test ~ especially before breakfast ~ try thinking of them as a your own Bryant Gumble and catch up on the morning news out there in the real world. You'll be surprised what opinions and arguments you can foment to take your mind off the medical proceedings.

Women ask me how I ever coped with losing my hair. I was prepared, that's how. Thanks to pre-treatment advice from a friend in remission I bought a good wig, long before I lost my hair. This gave the salesperson a chance to see the real me and to match my wig to my own color and hairstyle. It also gave me a chance to play with it, wear it, and make it a part of me before I had to.

Take a friend along for a second opinion. Mine told me I looked ten years younger! And take your checkbook ~ good wigs are not cheap but they're worth every cent. In many instances your health insurance will pick up part or all of the cost.

My wig is a Kanokelon, not real hair. It swizzles out, drips dry, and resets itself overnight. It's been a God send. I also bought a few more scarves and bandannas, the cotton kind. They stay on your head better than the silk and synthetic varieties.

I began to wonder before it all fell out, how silly I would look. I realized that there are other parts of my anatomy that I'd much rather hang onto, and they don't grow back if you lose them.

The long pains-taking process comes later. It takes forever for your hair to grow back so you can trim or style it, and many of us do not look our best, or even comfortable, with a pixie hair-do.

Don't be a turtle! I live in a small town, and being a teacher, am fairly well-known. Rumors breed in small towns. I decided the truth was far better to live with than rumors. I said, "I've had a cancer diagnosis," rather than "I've been ill." "I'm receiving chemotherapy," not "I'm being hospitalized." "I'm going for daily radiation." instead of "I'm having treatments."

You can be honest about how you feel, receiving visitors or refusing them. Well-wishers can act with honesty as well. The occasional probing busy-body can be handled with a wilting "Excuse me, but I'm very tired."

The hardest thing for me was recognizing that I needed help, and accepting it. I'm independent and somewhat of a loner. Depending on drivers to get me to daily radiation treatments an hour away, five days a week, for seven weeks, was a humbling experience. Folks set up a driving schedule. A fellow cancer patient and his wife offered to take me along. Neighbors called to do errands. A local grocery store delivered. My mailman picked up letters-to-go at the door. Friends and family took me shopping.

I learned to say "Yes, thank you, that would help," instead of "No, I'll be all right," when I really wasn't. It made the ordeals easier for all of us. People want to help. They need to be told what they can do, or when you would prefer that they stay away. In general, folks who have never dealt with cancer have no idea what to say or what to do. They feel helpless while wanting to be helpful. I was the same way, and so were you, before cancer entered our lives.

When remission comes, grapevine the good news! Everyone who helped you through it will feel as grand as you do and delighted to have been a part of that remission. Then the real joy comes when you feel well enough to be one of *them* and offer help to someone else.

You can make a difference for yourself and for others.

Fall 1992

Feeling Brighter

by Joyce Schwinn

Recently, a young man stood before an assemblage of University of Scranton students and began his speech by proclaiming "I'm not here because I'm dying of AIDS - I'm here because I'm LIVING with AIDS."

"That's it!" I said to myself. "That's the message that says it all for cancer patients: I'M NOT DYING OF CANCER. I'M LIVING WITH CANCER."

I, like millions of others, faced my cancer diagnosis with immediate thoughts of death. How long have I got? Will I be here for Christmas? Why plant the garden? Will I see the fringe tree bloom another year? (I took pictures of it, assuming it could be the last time I'd revel in its beauty.) And my kids, oh my kids; I'm not ready to leave them.

Doctors spoke of quality of life. I had no real idea what they meant, nor did they spell it out to me. Nor, I guess, did I ask. I considered, or at least my mind wandered through all sorts of awful options. Should I let it take its course and be done with it? I envisioned what the media unjustly has pictured: treatment more hellish than the disease.

Zombie-like, I wandered my house, unable to begin or finish any thought or task. I didn't sleep well. My family and friends clustered.

Finally, I decided to at least begin all the tests. At this point I learned to ask questions; a habit that stood me in good stead. Always I took a friend or relative with me, bless them, to help me remember the answers. They became, thank God, my care-givers. What a lovely and essential word that is!

My first support group was literally one phone call, set up by one of these care-giver friends. My support call came from a recent cancer survivor, who described symptoms, referred me to a wig shop, discussed medications and possible side-effects. These were all things my doctor could have answered, but I didn't know enough to ask. My new friend was very instrumental in my dealing with my first two chemotherapy treatments and their aftermath.

I was hospitalized for my chemo. Mine were long five day affairs. I learned not to rush home from the hospital. My recuperation was much smoother when I stayed longer. Thankfully, we now have Zofran, the wonderful new anti-nausea drug.

Cancer patients need to swap stories. With today's sophisticated medications, bewildering technology, and medical specialization, we need to find guidance in each other. It is almost as if we revert to grandmother's day of discussing catnip tea remedies over the backyard clothesline. We compare complicated prescriptions and sophisticated treatments instead of herbs and snake oil. We regenerate those herbs, holistic healing, and encouraging words. We exchange tales about symptoms, doctors, and care-giving.

We become aware, in ourselves and in the examples of others, of recovering; of still *being here;* marveling in feeling a little better, a little more able to cope. I call it "feeling brighter."

So here, a year later, I'm in remission. After all the talk, the questions, and the brighter feelings, I don't really know what remission means ~ and, again, no one spells it out. I know I'm me again, most of the time. I know my energy is returning. My feet are still numb but the rest of me works. Most of all, I'm looking forward; planning to teach again, to make music, and to do theater.

I guess that's what remission is. You can live with the feeling that any day, any symptom, it'll all start again. Or you can revel in the returning of your "old self" and plan some tomorrows. Maybe that's the quality of life the doctors couldn't explain a year ago. But then, a year ago I couldn't either.

Summer 1992

ELAINE SHUEY

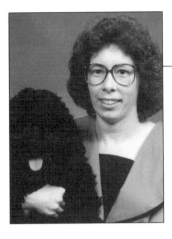

Elaine Shuey, who received her PhD from Kent State University in 1990, is a speech therapist and associate professor at East Stroudsburg University. She is happy to be back in the classroom with her students and to be able to enjoy her needlework projects, her assorted pets, and the menagerie of injured animals she cares for.

Tremendous Support

I was probably less surprised about getting breast cancer than most people. My mother, aunt, and great aunt all had it. However, I was surprised to be diagnosed at 36 years of age.

My mother had always reminded me of the importance of self-examinations and regular medical examinations. Her cancer was diagnosed early and she survived it with minimal medical treatment. I hoped the same would be true for me.

Initially, my major concern was who would care for my pets. My dog, Chop Shuey, was a particular concern. He's afraid of everyone and has a tendency to nip. My mother had died a few years earlier (of a heart attack, not cancer), so my dad came to my house to take care of things.

I teach at East Stroudsburg University and the spring 1993 semester had already started when I learned that I would need surgery. One of my colleagues suggested that I not tell my students why I was having surgery. However, I felt they would be more understanding and cooperative if they knew that this was something that couldn't be delayed. I was glad I told them. Students sent me cards and notes while I was in the hospital and when I returned home, which were tremendously uplifting, helpful, and humorous.

Convalescence was very boring. I like having time off but I've always had both housework and professional work to do. I couldn't handle the housework, and quickly caught up on the professional work that I could do. Even with over 50 channels, daytime television just wasn't for me. One day, I called my office-mate and asked her to measure her daughter so I could sew her an outfit. I finished that in one afternoon.

I looked forward to getting back to work and I returned to school exactly two weeks after surgery. I still couldn't put a shirt or sweater over my head because I couldn't raise my arms high enough. I found that I didn't own any button down shirts except some very fancy blouses. So, wearing a man's flannel shirt, I announced to my first class that they would be seeing a selection of shirts belonging to every male friend, both relatives and ex-boyfriends, I could borrow from. That issue became a running joke in class. When I failed to wear a green shirt on St. Patrick's Day, one student asked, "Don't you know any men who wear green shirts?" They also discussed whether pearls would enhance the femininity of the shirts. We all agreed they wouldn't. One of the students complimented me the first day I put a shirt over my head. I pointed out that I might have to wear it for days because I didn't think I could take it back over my head.

The honesty about my surgery and the jokes about the shirts made the transition back to school quite easy. Later in the semester, one student learned that her mother had breast cancer and another student had a breast cancer scare. Both felt free to talk to me about their fears and concerns. I was glad I had told them what was going on.

One of the things that I feared about this experience was that friends would back away. When my mother had cancer, one of her best friends didn't call, visit, or even send a card. I found that both close and casual friends rallied around me. One friend's mother, who had also had breast cancer, called me for a frank, open discussion that helped me to make some decisions.

1993 was a positive year for me. I survived cancer. I survived, when my little VW was totaled. I went to the pound and got a second dog who doesn't bite. I learned that I have some very good friends and a supportive family And I learned that, even if you miss a Dutot Museum meeting because you're having cancer surgery, someone will still put you in charge of a committee.

Fall 1995

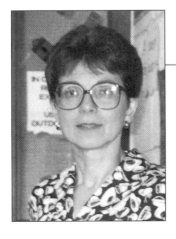

CYNTHIA STEVENS

Cynthia Stevens and her husband Curt, who is a five-year survivor of a bone marrow transplant for his non-Hodgkin's lymphoma, are both enthusiastic and energetic country-western dancers. Cynthia confesses that she continues her eternal quest for the perfect pair of dancing boots. She has been an elementary school teacher for 31 years, and says her students and her husband help her stay young and love life.

Who Cares For The Caregiver?

When a loved one receives a diagnosis of a life-threatening illness, you find yourself thrust into a new role ~ primary caregiver.

Most of us fill this role at different times and in different ways in our lives. However, now the caregiver role is pivotal in dealing with a formidable opponent ~ cancer.

When my husband, Curt, was diagnosed with non-Hodgkin's lymphoma seven years ago, we were both devastated. We thought we were doing everything right: good eating habits, exercise, and plenty of rest.

A diagnosis of cancer was an incredible shock to us. The best way to describe how we felt is that it "knocked the wind out of our sails."

Since then, we have been partners fighting this ill news. Cancer is a family affair. The patient is not the only one experiencing the disease.

These past years we have survived three bouts of chemotherapy, two of radiation, and a bone marrow transplant which took place four and a half years ago. We have had uphill battles and some defeats, but each of us has maintained a positive attitude and a sense of humor.

I firmly believe my role has been significant, for I chose to act as patient advocate for my husband. I had never heard of non-Hodgkin's lymphoma, but through extensive reading, and asking questions of doctors, nurses, and other lymphoma patients, I developed an understanding of this disease.

Curt did not want to know everything about his illness but I felt one of us needed to be knowledgeable so we would be better-equipped fighters. I continue to join him at doctors' appointments. I still take along my trusty little notebook in which I write any questions I'd like to have answered. No matter how insignificant the question may seem, I ask it. This I find gives me peace of mind.

The role of caregiver can be overwhelming at times. I have felt frightened, frustrated, angry, and exhausted. I have also felt great joy and hope. Often, it is lonely. Family and friends may ask about the patient but not about how you are doing. They sometimes forget that you, too, are experiencing this illness and life change.

Caregivers need to learn to care for themselves by utilizing methods that help them cope. You may be handling a full-time job and a family, and now you may have extra responsibilities in taking care of your home. Years ago a friend and I began a Caregivers' Support Group. I was able to express my fears and feelings to other caregivers who could identify with my experiences. I could receive comfort and give comfort, for we were all fighting together.

I began keeping a journal to express my feelings and thoughts ~ whatever they may be. This has been a tremendous release for me.

Curt and I have been involved with many different support groups for patients and their families through which we have developed special friendships.

We've had great moments of happiness as well as moments of sadness. Talking and sharing with others seems to be one of the most beneficial ways to cope with cancer. It may be difficult at first, for you are exposing your innermost thoughts, but it is certainly worth the effort.

I used to wonder whether our life would ever be the same as it was before cancer. It is not. But life is change. It does not stay the same. Besides, there have been so many positive things that have occurred because of cancer. It seems quite incredible but it is true.

I have discovered tremendous personal strength, spirit, and faith which I rarely tapped into before. Curt and I have learned to live life to the fullest day to day ~ and to fully enjoy our relationship. When you face death, your priorities change and being together becomes the most important goal.

We both have been blessed with wonderful families and friends who have supported us through our ups and downs.

I will continue to fight actively with Curt against this disease, and I will be certain to take care of myself ~ the caregiver.

Fall 1993

CAROLYN TETREAULT

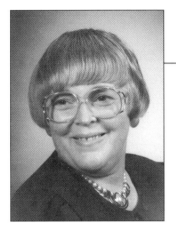

Carolyn Tetreault is a mental health worker at the Scranton Counseling Center and also enjoys her busy life with her husband of 35 years, Arthur, and their four children and five grandchildren. She is on the Board of Directors of the American Cancer Society and is the coordinator for the Reach for Recovery program which allows her to "touch another hand for helping, sharing and loving".

Reach for Recovery

A group of women who know and care, for they themselves have been there .

R - Is for the <u>RICHES</u> of each new day and our ability to show others there's still a way.

E - Is for the <u>ENTHUSIASM</u> God gave to you and me, and we as volunteers were meant to pass it on to others, just you wait and see.

A - Is for the <u>AVENUES</u> our life still has in store, it may not be easy, but should we ask for more?

C - Is for <u>COMMON SENSE</u>, to lend a helping hand, for giving of ourselves is part of God's great plan.

H - Is for the <u>HELPING</u> wherever there's a need, for life brings new growth by planting one small seed.

F - Is for <u>FORTUNATE</u> that we have another day to help one more woman along life's way.

O - Is for <u>OPENNESS</u> that two women can share, for you can only give if you've already been there.

R - Is for <u>REMEMBERING</u> we are not alone and there are many who may need us, for we do not journey alone.

R - Is for <u>RECOVERY</u> which we all need to share, for it helps us to get better just knowing someone is there.

E - Is for <u>EXCELLENCE</u> we can still have in life. Just give each day to God so he will remove the strife.

C - Is for the <u>COMING</u> days we do not know what is in store, but if we give of ourselves we will get so much more.

O - Is for <u>ONLY</u> and this one day, so try to make the most of it by sharing yourself along the way.

V - Is surely for <u>VICTORY</u> and all the battles that we have done, and by volunteering we can share with everyone.

E - Is for the <u>ENERGY</u> that comes from when we share, for it is never fun going it alone - it is better knowing someone is there.

R - Is for <u>REACHING</u> out, that all breast cancer women can do, for everyday may become like me and you.

Y - Is for the <u>YEARNING</u> that this dreaded disease could soon be beat.

So reach out in recovery and touch another hand for helping, sharing, and loving is the master's plan.

NRCI Editors Note: Reach For Recovery is an on-going program of the American Cancer Society. For more information call your local unit.

Fall 1995

LARRY THEILGARD

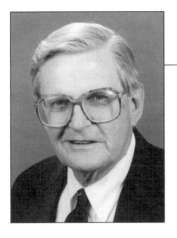

Larry Theilgard was diagnosed with prostate cancer in 1993 and was treated with a combination of radiation therapy and hormone therapy. He continues to take oral hormone therapy daily, and his cancer remains in complete remission. Now retired from his position as a vice president at Akzo-Nobel Salt, Inc., Larry is always ready and willing to talk with other men who have prostate cancer to explain both his medical and philosophical approach to this disease. Larry was a speaker at NRCI's 1994 *Survivors Celebration*.

Each Day Is a Special Gift

When I was a freshman in high school, I played the part of Wally Webb in Thornton Wilder's Pulitzer Prize winning play, "Our Town". The play left a lasting impression on me, especially the part where Wally's sister, Emily, who has died during childbirth, is granted her wish to return to earth for one day of her life. She selected her 16th birthday.

The scene depicts a close, happy family, but one so caught up in the hustle and bustle of daily life, they never stop to appreciate each other. Emily implores her family, as she revisits them, to open their eyes and hearts to one another, cherish and appreciate each day that they have together. She finally asks "Do human beings realize life while they live it?"

I have learned as a prostate cancer survivor, that each day is a special gift and the quality of life is more important than its quantity. Most of us take so much for granted, especially family and friends. We have so many days on this earth, and they slip away one by one. Every day that passes can never be replaced and missed opportunities to hug and say, "I care" are gone forever.

I have also learned from my illness that each individual is ultimately responsible for his or her own health. We owe it to ourselves and to our loved ones to be well informed on the important matters regarding healthy habits, nutrition, and treatments. Early detection of cancer is so important to improving chances of survival.

While survivorship is to be celebrated, we must not forget those who were not as fortunate and who have lost their brave fight against this illness. The courageous example many of these people have set for me I shall never forget.

Realizing that each day is a special gift, I have decided to live each day to its fullest. I have also learned to better appreciate a red streaked sky at sunset and the magic of a jewel bedecked starry night. What a wonderful way to get close to the Creator!

Always remember people do survive cancer, especially if it is detected early. Please promise me that you'll learn all you can about early detection, and if cancer is diagnosed, learn how to deal with it medically, emotionally, and nutritionally. And never underestimate the power of prayer.

Spring 1994

JILL TISCHLER

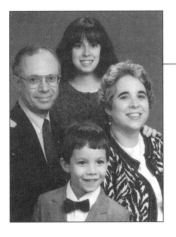

Jill Tischler underwent a bone marrow transplant for her breast cancer in 1995. Currently, she is gathering other cancer survivors' experiences for possible publication in order to help family and friends of people with cancer understand the trial of the disease. Jill hopes to be here as long as possible, and is fighting each day to do so. She hopes to be included in your prayers.

Still in the Picture

Though I am the seventh person in a row on my father's side of the family to develop cancer, my own diagnosis of breast cancer was still a shock. "Where do we go from here?" I asked, without tears, still groggy from the anesthesia administered for the biopsy. The second opinion came the next week, and the mastectomy followed a week later. My aunt lived for 29 years after her diagnosis of breast cancer, and I wanted to fight for the same chance.

The loss of my breast and impending baldness seemed almost unimportant. The thought of not being here to raise my children, aged 4 and 13, was intolerable. I could put my son to bed every night and help my daughter with her homework with only one breast. I'd do anything to stay alive.

In the hospital post-surgery, I felt like a poster child for breast cancer ~ somewhat foggy, but alive, walking, talking, visiting with family, and understanding why the surgery was vital. Three days post mastectomy, my oncologist announced: "Twelve nodes positive. It's not good. We're sending you for a bone marrow transplant." My mother, who did not understand this news, said that I turned as white as the hospital sheets. The fear and terror I felt seemed palpable. Bone marrow transplant? The phrase itself was terrifying.

I was definitely on the cancer express train.

Within two short weeks I'd been diagnosed with breast cancer, had a mastectomy, and had been told that I'd need a bone marrow transplant (BMT) very soon. As soon as I got home, I read everything I could about BMT, spoke to three women who had undergone the procedure, viewed a videotape (which turned out to be more terrifying than my own BMT experience), and started pressuring the insurance company and the staff at the hospital to please admit me immediately !

Undergoing a BMT is akin to having one's skin turned inside out. Throw in the risk of ebola-like effects caused by garden variety hospital germs, complete and helpless dependency on the most wonderful nurses, and feeling too weak to talk with my children by phone or even being allowed to see them for an entire month.

But a BMT is actually wonderful, because it can cure some very sick people. I think it might be apt to inscribe "All ye who enter here have no choice" over the door of the BMT ward.

I refused to hear anything negative while I was in the hospital. That included watching the news or anything else on TV. I spent every moment meditating or listening to audio tapes with healing messages. The regimen worked. My doctor called me the Nancy Kerrigan of the BMT ward, the silver medalist, because I was the second fastest engrafter of bone marrow they'd ever had. This taciturn, kind man who seemed to have put himself on a diet of very few words per day said, "Congratulations! You seemed to have dodged a lot of bullets. You didn't have a lot of the side effects that most people on this ward have had." I wrote this in my journal verbatim the moment he left the room.

My at-home post-transplant regimen of 100 days included wearing a surgical mask to prevent infection whenever I went outdoors, even in my own backyard, eating only canned fruits and vegetables instead of fresh foods, undergoing seven weeks of radiation, feeling exhausted, and remaining pretty much in isolation. The only time I left the house was for blood tests. Hospital staffers took one look at my scarf-swathed head and mask-covered face and just stared. "They think you're contagious," my mom said cheerfully.

One of the hardest facets of being ill is complete dependency on others. But my family was wonderful. My parents came from sunny Florida in December and stayed through April, despite my dad's health problems and his own need for care, and they helped with the children and the household. My mother came to Philadelphia with me and stayed in my hospital room 18 hours a day, holding my hand when the procedures left me too weak to talk. I often felt her strength kept me alive. I prayed that I'd outlive my parents, because they'd always said that losing a child was the greatest sorrow imaginable. I wanted to spare them such pain.

Although my husband wanted to spend lots of time with me in the hospital, it seemed vital for our children to have at least one parent at home. So he took on all of the "Mommy jobs" with the children, went to work, dealt with the insurance company almost daily, and wrote letters to our out-of-town friends and relatives.

Now I am at home and quite able to take care of my family, and that is what matters. Looking back, I realize how many people were wonderful to my family and me during this difficult time. A group of friends made dinner three times a week for three months. Friends drove my daughter to weekly piano and art lessons. A friend cared for my son every Saturday and sent a silver necklace with boxing gloves on it to symbolize my fight.

I received hundreds of cards and letters that were uplifting, supportive, and funny. People sent me Bernie Siegel books and tapes, pajamas, robes, flowers, a weekly copy of the Washington Post humor column, and a list of 100 funny movies to rent and view while recovering at home. Friends in our former home state gathered weekly and recited prayers for my recovery. A distant relative whom I've never met, who has undergone a liver transplant, wrote wonderfully inspiring letters which I read daily in the hospital. People respected my wishes for no phone calls ~ too draining ~ and sent notes instead.

It seems that when someone has cancer, family, friends, and co-workers want to help, but aren't always sure what to do or how to respond. They may confront their own mortality when someone close is seriously ill, and that is very scary for most people. The key seems to be to treat the person with cancer as the person you've always known, a person with multiple roles, interests and relationships. The person who is ill usually wants to look beyond the current experience to a healthy future.

The people who were the most helpful were those who dealt with their own emotions on their own time, and left me to deal with mine in my own way and time. My family, my three wonderful cousins who had been there before me, my terrific brother and sister, a few healthcare professionals, and my closest friends were all helpful emotionally.

People who were of the greatest assistance considered my practical needs, such as transporting my children, taking me to treatment appointments, or making hot dinners so my husband could keep working. They often showed up, unannounced, with food in hand. Others left dinner on the doorstep, rang the doorbell, and left. They performed, they didn't talk. Other people however, said, "Call me if there's anything I can do." I never called. I didn't have the energy and didn't want to impose.

Another aspect of being helpful, I think, is understanding the different phases a person with cancer experiences. I seemed to go through three phases. First, I needed information about the illness, treatment options, and possible side effects. Second, during and after my treatment, I was too sick or tired to interact. Third, during recovery, I wanted to get back to thinking about doing normal activities as my energy allowed. I would like to learn how others reacted to family and friends' attempts to help as I did or differently. I am gathering other cancer survivors' experiences for possible publication in order to help friends and family members of people with cancer know what to do and how to act. What did others do that helped lift your spirits or get you through treatment more easily? What do you wish others had done for you? What did others do that wasn't helpful? What do you think might help someone else? I hope to include personal interviews and questionnaire responses from cancer survivors. I know most cancer survivors have a story they would like to tell, and urge readers of *NewsNotes* to contact me with their stories:

Jill Tischler
P.O. Box # 1063
Kingston, PA 18704

Winter 1995

JUDY TUTINO

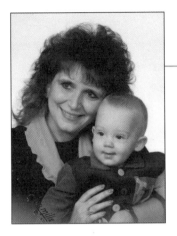

Judy Tutino sums up her life since her diagnosis of breast cancer three years ago as always keeping active, maintaining a positive attitude, and living life to the fullest. She manages to balance three full-time roles as a wife, mother, and registered nurse. She is vice president of marketing for a regional health services agency, assists her husband with their home-based business, and serves as a volunteer with several area health service organizations.

The Good Things in Life

Seven months after our first child was born, I was diagnosed with breast cancer. I had found a lump on my breast through self exam. What a traumatic experience! I had a brand new son who depended on me to take care of his every need. Now I had to juggle my life and take care of my special needs as well as my baby's.

After the devastating shock of my diagnosis subsided, I was overwhelmed by the care, love, and concern expressed by co-workers, friends, and most importantly my family, especially my husband and mother. They let me know I was not alone and that I could count on them at all times. I didn't realize how much I meant to them and how much they really mean to me.

I am a registered nurse, so when I was told I had breast cancer a multitude of questions and concerns ran through my mind. However, I had tremendous faith in my doctors. Dr. Scialla, Dr. Rostock, and Dr. Gallagher and all their staff were fantastic. They explained everything to me about my radiation and chemotherapy. They also kept me well informed about my particular case.

Through it all I kept a positive attitude. I am not going to say it was easy. It wasn't. I had a hard time at first dealing with my fears of the disease and of the treatments. But, I finally accepted my situation and decided I was going to beat this devastating disease.

I had a beautiful little boy, a wonderful, supportive husband, and a terrific family that I had to live for. I couldn't let cancer get me down.

I continued to work as Director of Community Services for Care, Inc. I took care of my baby, the house, did aerobics, was an Avon Representative, and a member of Bosom Buddies (a breast cancer support group). My mother was really special. Without her, I wouldn't have been able to accomplish all I did. She was always there to take care of the baby and to give me moral and psychological support.

I finally finished my treatments in June, 1993. I am trying to get back to a normal life again.

I look at life in a different light now. Somehow the things that seemed important before are not as important now. I appreciate life and everyone around me. I thank God every day for being with me and getting me through such a terrible ordeal. I pray each day that I have seen the last of my cancer so that I can concentrate on better and brighter things like ~ my son!

I personally appreciate and stress the importance of early detection. It can literally save your life.

Fall 1993

PHYLLIS VILLELLA

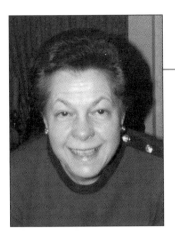

Phyllis Villella says that her diagnosis of cancer taught her to appreciate the special beauty of life, family, and friends. She retired from her job after her cancer treatment more than five years ago to devote more of her time to her personal interests including home decorating, gardening, reading, theater, and volunteer work.

It's Time for Some Reflection

Mark Twain was right. There are three forms of untruth, each one worse than the one before: lies, damned lies and statistics. Here I am five years after diagnosis, or as I tell my friends, five years past my "sell by" date. Statistically, my chances were poor for making it this far without a recurrence.

It's been quite an experience. What have I learned? What has this life-jolting experience taught me? Many things.

I learned the true meaning of positive thinking. I'm not referring to the advice to "think positive" glibly foisted upon you by well meaning friends who may really be advocating denial. No, that's not the kind of advice you

need. You learn to be patient and lovingly forgiving with people who want to change the subject when they hear the word cancer.

I learned that a positive attitude translates into positive action. You make and keep doctor's appointments as required; you take prescribed medications and treatments; you feel and express gratitude for the loving, supportive friends and family in your life; you turn to your faith to accept whatever the outcome may be; you revel in the beauty of nature and the world around you; you become willing to help another, even if it's being silent when you would like to complain about some distress you're feeling.

I've learned that chemotherapy and radiation can be your friends. I've developed a love-hate relationship with chemotherapy. I hate it for making me so terribly sick before it made me well, and for the devastating effect it has had on my body. But I love it for allowing me to continue with my life, even if it is in this somewhat compromised body.

I learned how important it is to stay involved with people, even if you're sick and weakened. I've learned what the expression "survivor's debt" means. You feel deeply motivated to pay back the blessings you've been given. I'll be paying that off for as long as I live.

As I close, I don't ever want to forget the valuable lessons cancer has taught me.

Spring 1994

FRANCIS M. WHITE

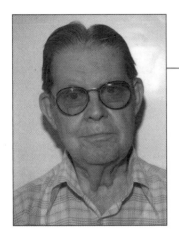

Francis White taught at the Philadelphia College of Pharmacy and Science for 42 years, and moved to the Poconos after retiring in 1983. He was diagnosed with cancer on Christmas Eve 1992. Today, he is thankful for his good health and to be able to enjoy life with his loving wife, their five children, and nine grandchildren.

Cancer Haiku

Check for Cancer NOW
Is the secret for success.
I'm a SURVIVOR!

How I licked Cancer
Requires regular checks NOW
For sure detection.

Early detection
Gives the doctor and you the
Best chance to win.

Now radiation
Or chemotherapy plays
Big role in treatment.

Trust in God and pray
The treatment will succeed and
You will live more days.

Note: HAIKU is an unrhymed Japanese poem of three lines containing 5,7,5 syllables respectively.

Winter 1995

Index